ALKALINE DIET cookbook for cancer

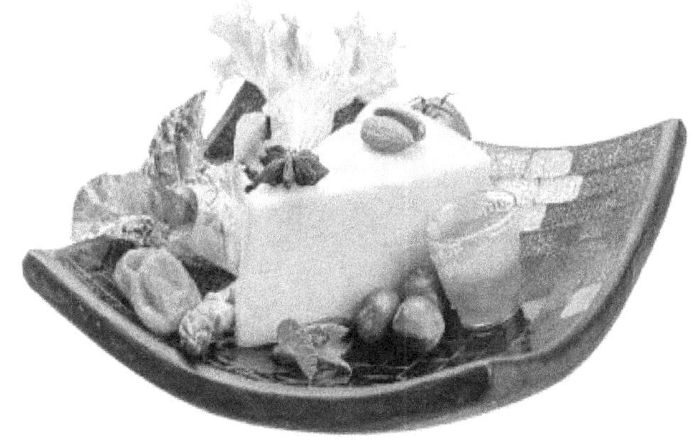

A Comprehensive Guide to Boosting Your Cancer Defense!

Dr. VIVIAN GREENE

Please scan the QR code to access additional books authored by Dr. Vivian Greene

Table of Contents

ABOUT THE AUTHOR

Dr. Vivian Greene is a highly regarded nutritionist and wellness specialist whose passion for promoting health and well-being through balanced and satisfying food choices has left an indelible mark on the world of nutrition. Her dedication to assisting individuals in achieving optimal health has made her a leading authority in the field of plant-based diets and nutrition.

With a doctorate in nutritional sciences, Dr. Greene possesses a deep understanding of the intricate relationship between food and health. Her extensive knowledge, coupled with her real-world experience, has solidified her reputation as a prominent expert in the field. Dr. Greene's mission is to inspire and educate individuals, helping them make transformative changes in their lives through informed dietary choices.

Throughout her career, Dr. Greene has authored numerous articles, academic papers, and best-selling books, sharing her expertise and insights on nutrition, plant-based diets, and meal planning. Her work is a testament to her commitment to empowering people to make healthier choices and lead vibrant, fulfilling lives.

Dr. Vivian Greene's unwavering dedication to improving the health and well-being of others has left an enduring legacy in the world of nutrition, making her a respected and influential figure in the field. Her work continues to inspire individuals to embrace a healthier lifestyle through informed dietary decisions.

Introduction

Hello and welcome to "The Alkaline Diet Cookbook: A Comprehensive Guide to Boosting Your Cancer Defense." One cannot stress the importance of diet in the fight against cancer and in bolstering one's health. This book is an all-inclusive guide designed to show you how the alkaline diet and your body's inherent defenses against cancer may work in extraordinary harmony.

Still, a powerful enemy, cancer affects people's lives all across the globe. Nevertheless, a growing corpus of scientific research highlights the critical role that pH balance and dietary decisions have in reducing the incidence of cancer and promoting overall well-being.

In this book, we explore in great detail the complex interactions between the alkaline diet and its significant effects on managing and preventing cancer. With a careful examination of scientific concepts, useful advice, and a wealth of delicious recipes, this book aims to empower you on your path to adopting an alkaline way of living

Deciphering the relationship between pH balance, cellular health, and the development of cancer, we negotiate the scientific terrain. We may take concrete steps to strengthen the body's defenses against cancer by modifying nutrition to create an alkaline environment. This is achieved by delving into the science behind acidity and alkalinity.

More than just a list of recipes, this book serves as a guide for achieving vitality. The basic principles of the alkaline diet are presented, giving you the information you need to make wise food decisions. We want to change people's perceptions about restricted diets by presenting them with mouthwatering meals that have been carefully chosen to strike a balance between gourmet enjoyment and alkalinity.

We also explore holistic lifestyle changes, acknowledging the synergistic effects of physical activity, stress reduction, and supplements in enhancing your body's anti-cancer defenses.

Words alone cannot express the joy, empowerment, and resiliency that these chapters contain. This book is designed to take you on a transforming journey toward health and vitality via professional insights, doable tactics, and motivational testimonies.

With any luck, this book will be a source of inspiration and information that will help you achieve a balance between perseverance in the face of hardship, health, and nutrition.

Understanding the Alkaline Diet

The idea behind the alkaline diet is to bring the pH levels of the body into a delicate equilibrium. Fundamentally, this dietary strategy prioritizes the eating of foods that support an alkaline environment above those that cause the body to become more acidic.

Recognizing the pH scale, which is a measurement of **acidity or alkalinity ranging from 0 to 14 with 7 being neutral, is essential to comprehending this diet.** For optimum health, the body normally functions in a slightly alkaline zone, or about pH 7.4.

This equilibrium is greatly impacted by the foods we eat. When digested, foods that generate an alkaline environment, such as fruits, vegetables, nuts, and legumes, have an alkalizing impact that helps to maintain or raise the pH levels in the body. On the other hand, meals high in acid, such as processed foods, meats, dairy products, and certain cereals, tend to reduce pH levels and may upset the body's normal balance.

Alkaline diet proponents claim that making a move to a more alkaline state may have several positive effects on health, such as increased energy, strengthened immunity, and a lower chance of developing certain chronic illnesses, including cancer.

Even though this dietary strategy has drawn attention, research is still being done to determine the scientific consensus about its actual influence on cancer prevention or therapy. While definitive data is still developing, several studies indicate that an alkaline diet may generate an environment less favorable to cancer development.

In the end, eating an alkaline diet means emphasizing entire, nutrient-dense foods that help the body maintain its normal pH equilibrium. This dietary change promotes general well-being by encouraging a thoughtful approach to eating in addition to emphasizing healthy choices.

In the chapters that follow, we'll examine the science behind the alkaline diet, discuss how it may help prevent cancer, and provide helpful advice on how to include alkaline foods in your regular meals.

Gaining an understanding of the alkaline diet is essential for maximizing its potential advantages. This book will help you navigate its complexities and make well-informed choices about your health and well-being.

What is the Alkaline Diet?

The foundation of the alkaline diet is the idea that certain meals may affect the pH levels of the body. It is often praised as a lifetime strategy rather than a temporary diet. Proponents recommend consuming fewer meals that are thought to be acid-forming and more foods that are thought to be alkaline-forming.

The basic idea is based on the pH scale, which is a scale from 0 to 14 that indicates how acidic or alkaline something is. The body aspires to balance, keeping its pH at around 7.4, which is slightly alkaline to promote optimum health. Our diets have an impact on this fragile equilibrium.

A diet rich in fruits, vegetables, nuts, seeds, legumes, and whole grains is usually considered alkaline-forming. After being digested, these meals leave behind alkaline residues that may help raise or maintain the pH levels in the body.

On the other hand, a lot of processed foods, meats, dairy products, refined sugars, and certain cereals are foods that cause acidity. After digestion, these meals might leave the body with an acidic residue that could upset the proper alkaline balance.

With an emphasis on plant-based, nutrient-dense meals and their function in maintaining the body's natural pH balance, the alkaline diet encourages a change in eating habits. This dietary strategy promotes attention to overall nutrition and its effects on health in addition to advocating for particular food choices.

The scientific evidence for the health advantages of an alkaline diet, such as increased energy, better digestion, and less inflammation, is still developing, despite the claims made by supporters. There is still much to learn about the possible effects of nutrition on diseases like cancer prevention.

The alkaline diet, which emphasizes the eating of complete, unprocessed foods that support an alkaline environment inside the body, essentially acts as a guideline for making educated dietary decisions. Gaining an understanding of the subtleties of this diet plan is the first step towards incorporating its ideas into your everyday routine.

This book will cover the science of the alkaline diet, and how it relates to cancer prevention, and provide helpful tips and recipes to help you incorporate these ideas into your cooking.

Knowing what the alkaline diet entails can help you take advantage of its possible health benefits and make well-informed choices about your diet and general health.

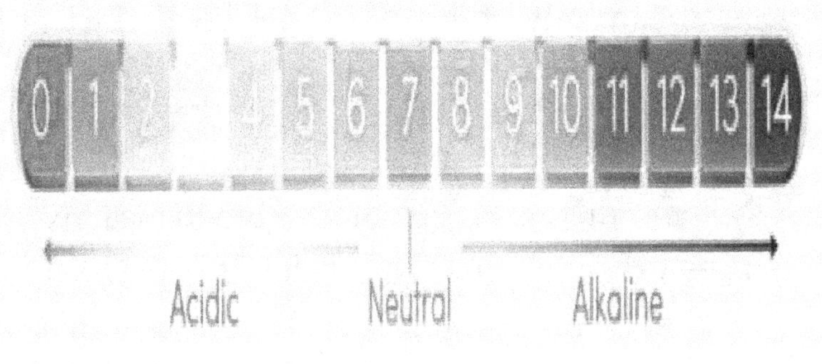

How pH Balance Affects Health

The measurement of acidity or alkalinity in the body, or pH balance, is essential for preserving good health and normal physiological processes. The equilibrium between positively charged (acid-forming) and negatively charged (alkaline-forming) ions found in biological fluids and tissues is referred to as the body's pH level.

Many physiological functions, including enzyme activity, cellular metabolism, and the body's capacity to fight illness, depend on a pH balance. To make sure these activities run as smoothly as possible, the body carefully controls the pH levels in its tissues within a certain range.

The ideal pH ranges for various body systems differ. For example, blood usually has a pH of 7.35 to 7.45, which is somewhat alkaline. Any notable departure from this range has the potential to impair vital processes and cause health problems.

Overly acidic or alkaline pH levels in the body may affect cellular processes, enzyme activity, and the body's natural defensive systems. The body may use alkaline supplies, including calcium from bones, to counteract an overly acidic environment. This might eventually have an impact on bone health.

Furthermore, an unbalanced pH environment might make it more difficult for the body to effectively cleanse and get rid of waste. Numerous health concerns, including exhaustion, gastrointestinal disorders, compromised immune systems, and heightened vulnerability to certain illnesses, may be caused by this.

Although the body has strong systems in place to maintain pH equilibrium, lifestyle, and food choices may have an impact. The pH levels of our bodies are greatly influenced by the meals we eat, with foods that create alkaline frequently supporting a more balanced pH than those that form acid.

Making thoughtful food decisions is crucial, as shown by the complex interplay between pH balance and health. Eating a diet high in foods that generate an alkaline environment may help preserve the body's natural pH balance, which promotes general health and vigor.

We'll go into more detail on how eating, and the alkaline diet in particular affects pH balance and possible health effects in the parts that follow, including how it may help prevent cancer.

Understanding the significant impact pH balance has on health establishes the foundation for investigating how to maximize it via food choices and lifestyle adjustments.

Alkaline Diet and Cancer: Exploring the Connection

For a long time, both scientists and health enthusiasts have been fascinated by the connection between nutrition and cancer. The alkaline diet has drawn interest in this field of study due to its potential for managing and preventing cancer.

The main goal of the alkaline diet is to consume more foods that generate an alkaline state while consuming fewer items that form an acidic one. Advocates of this dietary strategy believe that a more alkaline internal environment may reduce the risk of cancer initiation or progression.

Though fascinating, the findings of scientific examinations exploring the relationship between nutrition, pH balance, and cancer are still equivocal. Although some research indicates that an alkaline environment may slow the development of cancer cells or lower the chance of developing specific types of cancer, this is still early data that needs further investigation.

An alkaline diet's possible protection against cancer has been explained in part by how it affects cellular health. Since cancer cells grow best in acidic settings, proponents of the alkaline diet suggest that circumstances for cancer cell proliferation may be lessened by altering dietary choices to create a more alkaline milieu.

Furthermore, the focus of an alkaline diet on whole, plant-based foods high in antioxidants, vitamins, and minerals may improve general health and strengthen the body's defenses against cancer.

It's crucial to remember that, even if dietary interventions—such as the alkaline diet—may help prevent cancer or assist existing cancers, they shouldn't be seen as stand-alone therapies. They need to be included in all-inclusive healthcare programs that include appropriate medical advice, care, and lifestyle modifications.

The area of science is always changing when it comes to comprehending the complex link between nutrition, pH balance, and cancer. Current investigations are being conducted to clarify the precise processes that underlie this relationship and determine the practical implications for cancer prevention and supportive care.

The goal of investigating the link between the alkaline diet and cancer is to provide a more comprehensive knowledge of the impact of nutrition on health. It emphasizes the need for continuing research and the demand for an all-encompassing strategy for managing and preventing cancer.

Chapter 1

CANCER AND pH BALANCE

Phenomenological discussions and investigations into the potential impact of pH levels on the initiation and spread of cancer have been sparked by the correlation between cancer and the body's pH balance.

In their microenvironment, cancer cells show distinctive features; in contrast to healthy tissues, they often create a slightly acidic milieu. Through mechanisms that facilitate their multiplication and help them elude the body's natural defenses, it is thought that this acidic environment supports cancer cell growth and survival.

Even in the presence of oxygen, cancer cells prefer to use glycolysis, a process that creates energy in the absence of oxygen. This phenomenon is known as the Warburg effect. The tumor microenvironment becomes more acidic as a result of this metabolic change, which also increases lactic acid generation.

Yet, the exact cause of cancer is still unknown and has many facets, even though an acidic environment is linked to the disease's development. It is vital to understand that the body performs a variety of physiological functions at a highly controlled pH equilibrium and that variables other than nutrition may cause departures from this balance.

Theories about the alkaline diet's possible effects on cancer have surfaced because of its emphasis on creating an alkaline environment inside the body. An alkaline diet high in fruits, vegetables, and other items that promote an alkaline environment may help reduce the development of cancer cells, according to proponents.

It is still a topic of continuous scientific inquiry to determine if pH balance directly affects cancer. Though some research indicates links between acidic surroundings and the development of cancer, more thorough scientific research is needed to substantiate these results before they can be used to guide dietary choices or treatment approaches.

Navigating intricate biological mechanisms and their consequences for the course of illness is necessary to comprehend how cancer and pH equilibrium interact. Comprehending dietary and lifestyle variables as part of an integrated strategy for cancer prevention and treatment is crucial when approaching this connection, as is maintaining a thorough awareness of cancer biology.

The Science Behind pH and Cancer

Scientific research has examined the connection between pH levels and cancer, highlighting the potential impact of the body's pH balance on the growth and behavior of cancer cells.

The pH scale, which goes from 0 to 14 and has 7 as neutral, is used to measure acidity or alkalinity. Body fluids have an alkaline pH of around 7.4, which the body tries to maintain to support numerous physiological processes and optimum cellular function.

A microenvironment produced by cancer cells is often more acidic than the surrounding healthy tissues. It is believed that by promoting mechanisms that enable cell proliferation, invasion, and immune system evasion, this acidic environment accelerates the advancement of cancer.

The altered metabolism of cancer cells is one of the reasons contributing to the acidic conditions in the tumor microenvironment. The metabolic adaption known as the Warburg effect, which is present in many cancer cells, causes an increase in lactic acid production and adds to the acidic environment around the tumor.

Signaling pathways that control cell growth and survival may be influenced by acidic environments, which might encourage cancer cells' aggressive nature.

Although there is evidence linking acidic surroundings to the advancement of cancer, the precise causal connection between acidity levels and cancer is still unclear. Beyond pH balance, many genetic, environmental, and lifestyle variables contribute to the complexity of cancer.

The idea behind the alkaline diet is that by eating foods that increase the body's alkalinity, one may be able to inhibit the development of cancer cells. This diet plan seeks to balance pH levels by focusing on foods that generate an alkaline environment, such as fruits, vegetables, and certain grains.

Research on how an alkaline diet affects cancer is still in progress. Although some studies point to links between dietary habits and the risk of cancer, further investigation is required to confirm these results and convert them into evidence-based dietary recommendations.

Gaining knowledge about the scientific foundations of pH and its possible impact on cancer may help one better understand the complex interactions between cellular environments and the development of illness. It draws attention to the need for a thorough investigation and an all-encompassing strategy for cancer prevention and treatment.

The investigation of the relationship between pH and cancer highlights the complexity of cancer biology and the continuous effort to understand its processes, providing hints about possible directions for integrative health methods.

pH Levels and Cellular Health

Sustaining ideal pH levels is essential for the well-being of cells and the effective operation of the human body. The pH scale is a vital tool for establishing an environment that is favorable to cellular activity since it quantifies a substance's acidity or alkalinity.

The basic building blocks of life, cells, rely greatly on a pH environment that is balanced for their proper functioning. To sustain cellular operations, enzyme activity, and vital biochemical processes, the body maintains pH levels within a certain range.

Every cell has an ideal pH range for optimum operation. pH variations affect many biological functions, such as protein synthesis, metabolism, and the passage of nutrients and waste materials across cell membranes.

The equilibrium of cells may be upset by an imbalance in pH values, either toward acidity or alkalinity. Cellular processes may be affected in an acidic environment, which might result in changes to enzyme activity, a decrease in energy generation, and a higher vulnerability to cellular harm.

On the other hand, a more alkaline environment may promote cellular health by maintaining cellular integrity, promoting effective nutrient absorption, and offering the ideal conditions for enzymatic processes.

The body uses several processes to maintain the pH equilibrium. The lungs, kidneys, and other organs collaborate with different buffering systems to maintain the proper pH values in body fluids and tissues.

Nonetheless, outside variables including nutrition and lifestyle decisions may affect pH levels. For example, the alkaline diet places a strong emphasis on eating foods that generate an alkaline environment in the body. This dietary strategy emphasizes plant-based, high-nutrient meals that complement the pH balance of the body to promote cellular health.

Science research never stops investigating the connection between cellular health and pH levels. Although keeping pH at its ideal level is vital, it's essential to remember that the body's systems are skilled at doing so and that little variations often don't immediately pose a danger to health.

Knowing how pH affects cellular health emphasizes how important it is to make wise food and lifestyle decisions. Optimizing pH levels and fostering cellular vitality may be achieved by providing the body with a well-balanced, nutrient-rich food and encouraging a healthy lifestyle.

The investigation of pH levels and cellular health sheds light on the complex interplay between the internal environment and cellular processes, highlighting the need to maintain a balanced internal environment for maximum cellular viability.

Acidic Environments and Cancer Growth

The tumor microenvironment, which is the habitat for cancer cells and helps them multiply, is often more acidic than the surrounding healthy tissues. It is thought that this acidic environment in the tumor microenvironment is a major factor in the development and spread of cancer.

Acidity develops in the tumor microenvironment due to several reasons, including cancer cells' altered metabolic metabolism. Many cancer cells exhibit the Warburg effect, which increases dependence on glycolysis—a process that generates energy in an oxygen-poor environment—leading to the buildup of lactic acid and the consequent acidification of the surrounding environment.

The tumor microenvironment's acidic conditions may have a variety of impacts that aid in the spread of cancer. First off, an acidic environment may encourage cancer cells' invasive tendency, making it easier for them to metastasize to far-off locations inside the body and spread to nearby tissues.

Moreover, signaling pathways linked to cancer cell survival, proliferation, and resistance to cell death processes may be impacted by acidic environments. These acidic conditions cause cancer cells to adapt, which may make them more aggressive and resistant to traditional treatments.

Acidic environments may also affect the immune system in the tumor microenvironment, which might weaken the body's defenses against cancerous cells. This changed immune response may foster an environment that is more conducive to the survival and growth of cancer cells.

Though there is evidence linking acidic surroundings to the development of cancer, the precise causal connection is still unclear and the topic of continuing study. Beyond pH levels, a variety of variables, including genetic abnormalities, environmental conditions, and lifestyle factors, may impact the complex illness known as cancer.

Clarity on the complex connections between cancer cells and their environments is provided by an understanding of the effects of acidic environments on cancer progression. It emphasizes how crucial it is to investigate treatment techniques that attempt to disrupt the tumor microenvironment, such as those that modify pH levels, to stop the spread of cancer.

Scientists are working to identify the processes by which acidity affects the progression of cancer. This research is continuing. This research may open the door to novel cancer therapy approaches that focus on the distinct characteristics of the tumor microenvironment.

Investigating acidic surroundings and how they contribute to the development of cancer is an important field of study in understanding the intricacies of cancer biology. It highlights the need for cutting-edge treatment approaches meant to sabotage the favorable circumstances inside the tumor microenvironment that promote the growth of cancer.

Alkalinity as a Defense Against Cancer

The theory behind using alkalinity as a cancer defense is that making the body's milieu more alkaline might impede the development and spread of cancer cells.

It is thought that alkalinity, which is often linked to a pH balance that is just over 7, reduces the conditions that support the survival and growth of cancer cells. This theory is based on data indicating that cancer cells prefer acidic environments and have difficulty proliferating in alkaline surroundings.

This theory's proponents believe that an alkaline environment may prevent cancer from growing via several different processes. First, it has been suggested that an alkaline environment might hinder cancer cells' capacity to spread and infiltrate neighboring tissues, therefore delaying the course of the illness.

Moreover, cancer cells may be more vulnerable to therapies like radiation and chemotherapy in an alkaline environment. It is hypothesized that by changing the pH equilibrium, these therapies may be more successful in making cancer cells susceptible to them.

Also, a strong immune response is believed to be supported by an alkaline environment, which may strengthen the body's defenses against cancer cells. A pH-balanced environment may help maintain proper immune function by making it harder for cancer cells to proliferate.

While the idea of alkalinity as a cancer defense is fascinating, there is currently a lack of scientific data to support alkalinity's direct influence on cancer prevention or therapy. The impact of pH balance on cancer is still being investigated, and more thorough research is needed to validate these findings.

The goal of the alkaline diet is to encourage the body to become more alkaline by emphasizing the intake of foods that generate an alkaline environment, such as fruits, vegetables, and certain grains. Although many people who want to improve their health use this dietary strategy, further research is needed to determine how directly it affects cancer prevention or treatment.

Gaining knowledge about alkalinity's possible significance as a cancer-prevention strategy will help one better understand the intricate interactions between body chemistry and cancer biology. Even if the theory is fascinating, it's important to view this idea critically, acknowledging that the battle against cancer requires thorough study and evidence-based tactics.

Research efforts are underway to clarify the processes behind the impact of pH balance on cancer biology, as scientific knowledge grows. This investigation could lead to the discovery of cutting-edge therapeutic approaches that use the pH balance of the body to enhance current cancer therapies.

The analysis of alkalinity as a possible cancer defense represents a promising field of study, providing insights into novel strategies that might aid in the continuous fight against this complicated illness.

Chapter 2

GETTING STARTED WITH THE ALKALINE DIET

Starting an alkaline diet entails adopting a food strategy aimed at encouraging an alkaline environment in the body. Making the switch to this lifestyle means progressively eating more meals that generate an alkaline stomach while ingesting less items that form an acidic stomach.

Principles of the Alkaline Diet

The alkaline diet is based on the idea that certain meals may affect the pH levels of the body. Its goal is to preserve or enhance a slightly alkaline environment for general health and wellbeing. This dietary strategy places a strong emphasis on eating foods that increase alkalinity and minimizes the intake of items that make the body more acidic.

Alkaline Foods vs. Acidic Foods

One of the main tenets of the alkaline diet is the division of foods into acidic and alkaline groups. Recognizing these differences enables people to make educated dietary decisions that are meant to encourage a more alkaline environment in the body.

Foods That Form Alkaline

Foods that leave the body with alkaline residues after metabolism are known as alkaline-forming foods. Usually, they are linked to encouraging a more alkaline pH equilibrium. Foods that generate an alkaline environment include:

Fruits: Melons, berries, citrus fruits (oranges and lemons), and most other fruits (cranberries excepted).

Vegetables include leafy greens (kale, spinach), cruciferous (broccoli, cauliflower), root vegetables (beets, carrots), and other veggies like bell peppers and cucumbers.

Nuts and Seeds: Raw almonds, sunflower seeds, pumpkin seeds, and most other nuts and seeds.

Legumes: Peas, beans, and lentils are often regarded as alkaline-forming foods.

<u>Foods That Form An Acid</u>

Foods that produce acidic residues in the body after digestion are referred to as acid-forming foods. These meals are thought to increase the body's acidity. Foods that might cause acid reflux include:

Animal Proteins: Generally speaking, fish, poultry, eggs, and meats are acid-forming foods.

Dairy Products: Foods containing dairy, such as cheese, yogurt, and milk.

Processed Foods: A lot of convenience foods, packaged snacks, refined sweets, and processed grains may all cause acidity.

Some Grains: According to some dietary theories, certain grains, such as wheat, oats, and rice, may create acids.

Alkaline and Acidic Food Equilibrium

To maintain or encourage a more alkaline pH inside the body, the alkaline diet advocates for a larger consumption of foods that generate an alkaline rather than an acidic equilibrium. It is preferable to achieve a balance that tends toward alkalinity rather than eliminating substances that cause acidity.

One of the main components of the alkaline diet is the categorization of foods as acidic or alkaline, however, it's important to remember that the body's pH balance is closely controlled by several physiological processes. The effect of certain meals on pH levels generally may vary from person to person and may not be the only factor influencing overall health outcomes.

Making dietary decisions that are in keeping with the alkaline diet's tenets is made easier when one is aware of the differences between foods that generate an acidic environment and those that do not. Overall health and well-being may be supported by eating a range of nutrient-dense, alkaline-forming meals while reducing acidic-forming ones.

Creating an Alkaline Environment in Your Body

The goal of the alkaline diet is to create an internally alkaline environment, or apH balance that is thought to promote optimum health and vitality. Although the body has its systems for maintaining pH balance, proponents of the alkaline diet recommend modifying one's food and lifestyle to promote an alkaline condition.

1. Place a Focus on Alkaline-Forming Foods

Eat a wide variety of fruits and vegetables, but focus on leafy greens, cruciferous vegetables, and vibrant fruits like berries, which are generally alkaline-forming.

Nuts and Seeds: Add unprocessed, raw almonds, pumpkin seeds, chia seeds, and other nuts and seeds.

Legumes: Since beans, lentils, and peas are often thought of as alkaline-forming foods, include them in your meals.

2. Cut Back on Foods That Form Acid

Limit Animal Proteins: Since meats, poultry, fish, and eggs often cause the body to become acidic, consume them in moderation.

Reduce Your Intake of Processed and Refined Meals: Refined grains, sugary snacks, and processed meals all tend to increase acidity.

Think About Acidic Foods: Try to limit your consumption of some grains and dairy products as part of a balanced diet.

3. Drinking Alkaline Beverages to Hydrate

Alkaline Water: To enhance hydration and maybe contribute to alkalinity, think about drinking alkaline water, which is often enhanced with minerals or modified to a higher pH level.

Lemon Water: It is said that consuming lemon-infused water or adding lemon to your water would have an alkalizing impact on your body.

4. Conscious Eating Practices

Maintain a balanced intake of foods that create acids and alkaloids by practicing portion control.

Chew Your Meal: Give your meal a good chewing motion to help with digestion and nutritional absorption. This may also help the body maintain pH equilibrium.

5. Harmonize with Lifestyle Elements

Exercise regularly: Physical exercise is often linked to general health and may support initiatives to keep the interior environment in harmony.

Stress management: Since stress may affect one's general health, including pH balance, include stress-reduction strategies like yoga, meditation, or mindfulness exercises.

Although the alkaline diet encourages food modifications and lifestyle adjustments that create an alkaline environment in the body, it's important to approach these changes with a balanced mindset. The complicated control of pH in the body is not just dependent on nutrition.

It may be possible to promote general health and well-being by implementing healthy lifestyle practices and eating a diet high in alkaline-forming plant-based foods. Individual reactions to dietary adjustments might differ, so it's best to speak with medical specialists before making big dietary changes.

Comprehending the fundamentals of establishing an alkaline milieu inside the body provides valuable perspectives on plausible dietary and lifestyle modifications that might be by the objectives of the alkaline diet, which are to encourage a more alkaline internal milieu.

Tips for Transitioning to an Alkaline Diet

Making incremental, deliberate dietary adjustments is necessary to shift to an alkaline diet. The following advice will help you accept the alkaline diet's tenets and facilitate the transition:

1. Get Started Slowly

Start by progressively increasing the amount of foods that create an alkaline diet and decreasing the amount of foods that make an acidic diet. A more seamless and long-lasting transition may result from this incremental change.

2. Accept a Variety of Vegetables and Fruits

Try a variety of fruits and vegetables, particularly those with vibrant colors and lush greens. Try experimenting with various recipes to creatively include them in your meals.

3. Give Plant-Based Proteins Top Priority

Investigate plant-based protein sources such as quinoa, tofu, tempeh, and legumes (beans, lentils). These may be great substitutes for animal proteins.

4. Careful Meal Preparation

To guarantee a balanced intake of alkaline-forming foods throughout the day, plan your meals. Include a variety of dietary categories, but prioritize foods that are high in alkalinity.

5. Choose Complete, Natural Foods

Select whole grains rather than processed ones, such as buckwheat, millet, and quinoa. When it comes to snacking or meal additions, go for raw, unprocessed nuts and seeds.

6. Learn About Alkaline Drinks

Investigate alkaline drinks such as alkaline water, green tea, and herbal teas. Try adding citrus fruits, such as lime or lemon, to water to create a cool, perhaps alkalizing beverage.

7. Carefully read the labels

Keep an eye out for minimally processed meals with identifiable components by reading food labels. Seek alternatives that follow the guidelines of the alkaline diet.

8. Discover Through Alkaline Recipes

Explore and test out recipes for an alkaline diet found in cookbooks or internet sites. This may complement alkaline principles while bringing excitement and diversity to your meals.

9. Maintain Hydration

Make drinking water a priority and try to consume the most possible throughout the day. Think about adding lemon or alkaline-infused water to your daily hydration regimen.

10. Listen to your own body.

Observe your body's reaction to food modifications. Since every person's body is different, pay attention to how you feel and modify your diet appropriately.

11. Seek Advice When Necessary

For individualized direction and assistance, consider speaking with a nutritionist or other healthcare practitioner who is familiar with the alkaline diet.

Making small, lasting modifications to your eating habits is the key to switching to an alkaline diet. Accept the trip, put balance first, concentrate on adding more nutrient-dense, alkaline-forming foods, and keep your general health and well-being in mind.

Alkaline Foods and Their Benefits

Essential elements of an alkaline diet are alkaline foods, meaning they digest and leave behind an alkaline residue. These foods are linked to many health advantages and are thought to promote an internally alkaline environment.

1. Packed with Nutrients

Fruits and Vegetables: Rich in vitality-promoting vitamins, minerals, antioxidants, and phytonutrients, fruits and vegetables that generate an alkaline environment are also great sources of these nutrients. They boost the body's natural defensive mechanisms and encourage the health of cells.

2. Promotes Equilibrium pH

Alkaline-forming meals try to bring the body's pH levels back into balance, which may help to create an environment that is more alkaline inside. It is thought that this equilibrium promotes general health and ideal cellular performance.

3. Inflammatory-Reduction Capabilities

Reduction of Inflammation: An abundance of alkaline foods, particularly leafy greens, cruciferous vegetables, and certain fruits, have anti-inflammatory qualities that may aid in the body's reduction of inflammation.

4. Nutritional Status

Helps with Digestion: Fruits, vegetables, and legumes are high-fiber, alkaline foods that help with normal digestion, regularity, and the development of a healthy gut microbiota.

5. Improved Drinking Water

Alkaline Beverages: Some alkaline drinks, such as lemon-infused water or alkaline water, may help with improved hydration and hence promote general health and well-being.

6. Possible Control of Weight

Meals Rich in Nutrients but Low in Calories: Alkaline meals are often rich in nutrients but low in calories. When included in a balanced diet, increasing the amount of foods that generate an alkaline state may aid in good weight control.

7. Higher Levels of Energy

Vitality and Energy: Rich in nutrients, alkaline foods may help boost energy levels and improve general well-being by giving the body the nutrition it needs to perform at its best.

8. Protection Against Oxidants

Rich in Antioxidants: A lot of foods that generate an alkaline stomach are high in antioxidants, which assist in scavenging free radicals, shielding cells from harm, and maybe reduce the chance of developing certain chronic illnesses.

9. Possible Assistance for Bone Health

Calcium-Rich Foods: Leafy greens and certain nuts are examples of alkaline foods that are rich in calcium. Bone health and density are supported by an adequate calcium intake.

10. Advantages for Heart Health

Heart-Healthy Nutrients: A diet high in alkaline foods, such as certain fruits, vegetables, nuts, and seeds, may help promote cardiovascular health since they are high in heart-healthy nutrients including fiber, potassium, and healthy fats.

Including a selection of foods that generate an alkaline environment in your diet may have many health advantages. While more research is needed to confirm the direct effects of an alkaline diet on certain health outcomes, eating a diet high in nutrient-dense, alkaline foods may improve general health and well-being.

List of Alkaline Foods

Fruits

- Lemons
- Limes
- Oranges
- Grapefruits
- Berries (strawberries, blueberries, raspberries)
- Apples
- Watermelon
- Cantaloupe
- Kiwi
- Cherries

Vegetables

- Spinach
- Kale
- Swiss chard
- Broccoli
- Cauliflower
- Cabbage
- Brussels sprouts

- Bell peppers
- Celery
- Cucumber
- Zucchini

Leafy Greens

- Arugula
- Romaine lettuce
- Collard greens
- Bok choy
- Beet greens
- Dandelion greens

Root Vegetables

- Carrots
- Beets
- Sweet potatoes
- Radishes
- Turnips

Legumes

- Lentils
- Chickpeas

- Black beans
- Kidney beans
- Pinto beans

Nuts and Seeds (Raw and Unsalted)

- Almonds
- Walnuts
- Chia seeds
- Flaxseeds
- Pumpkin seeds
- Sunflower seeds

Whole Grains

- Quinoa
- Millet
- Buckwheat
- Amaranth

Others

- Tofu
- Tempeh
- Seaweed

- Herbal teas (chamomile, peppermint)
- Alkaline water (high pH water)

Incorporating a diverse range of these alkaline-forming foods into your meals can contribute to a balanced and nutrient-rich diet. It's essential to note that the classification of foods as alkaline or acidic is based on certain dietary philosophies and may not reflect the food's pH impact in the body. Always consult a healthcare professional before making significant dietary changes.

Recipes and Meal Plans

1. Alkaline Green Smoothie

Ingredients:

- ❖ 2 cups leafy greens (spinach, kale)
- ❖ 1 cucumber
- ❖ 1 green apple
- ❖ ½ lemon (peeled)
- ❖ 1-inch piece of ginger
- ❖ 1 cup coconut water

Instructions:

- Blend all ingredients until smooth.
- Add more water for desired consistency.

2. Quinoa Veggie Bowl

Ingredients:

- ❖ 1 cup cooked quinoa
- ❖ 1 cup mixed veggies (bell peppers, broccoli, carrots)
- ❖ ½ cup chickpeas

- ❖ 2 tablespoons lemon juice
- ❖ 1 tablespoon olive oil
- ❖ Herbs and spices (oregano, thyme, garlic powder)

Instructions:

- ❖ Sauté veggies and chickpeas in olive oil and spices.
- ❖ Mix in cooked quinoa and lemon juice.
- ❖ Serve with a side of leafy greens.

Alkaline Diet Meal Plan (Sample)

Day 1:

Breakfast: Alkaline green smoothie

Lunch: Quinoa veggie bowl

Dinner: Baked salmon with steamed broccoli and a mixed greens salad

Day 2:

Breakfast: Chia seed pudding topped with berries

Lunch: Lentil soup with a side of mixed greens

Dinner: Stir-fried tofu with bok choy and brown rice

Day 3:

Breakfast: Overnight oats with almond milk, topped with sliced bananas and nuts

Lunch: Chickpea salad with spinach, bell peppers, and a lemon-tahini dressing

Dinner: Roasted vegetable medley (zucchini, carrots, and beets) with quinoa

Tips for Alkaline Diet Meal Planning

Variety is Key: Incorporate a diverse range of alkaline-forming foods in each meal to ensure a broad spectrum of nutrients.

Balance Macronutrients: Aim for a balance of carbohydrates, healthy fats, and plant-based proteins in your meals.

Meal Prep: Plan and prepare meals in advance to stay consistent with alkaline choices throughout the week.

Hydration: Ensure adequate water intake and consider adding alkaline water or lemon-infused water to your routine.

Snack Smart: Opt for alkaline snacks like raw nuts, fresh fruits, or veggies with hummus.

Creating recipes and meal plans aligned with the alkaline diet involves incorporating plenty of fruits, vegetables, nuts, seeds, and whole grains while minimizing processed foods and acidic-forming choices. Adjust recipes based on personal preferences and consult with a healthcare professional for personalized guidance.

Chapter 3

ALKALINE RECIPES FOR CANCER DEFENSE

Alkaline Breakfast Recipes for Cancer Defense

Bonus 60 days Meal Plan and Template

Alkaline Green Smoothie Bowl

INGREDIENTS

1. 2 cups spinach
2. 1 ripe avocado
3. 1 banana
4. 1 cup almond milk
5. 1 tablespoon chia seeds

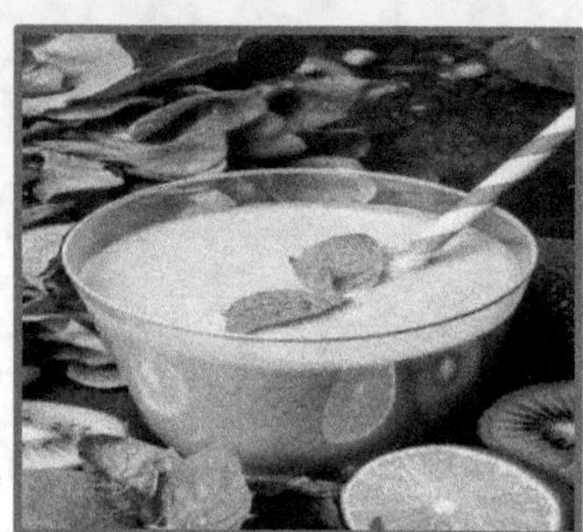

INSTRUCTIONS

1. Blend spinach, avocado, banana, and almond milk until smooth.
2. Pour into a bowl, top with chia seeds, and enjoy!

NUTRITION PER SERVING

- ❖ *Calories: 280*
- ❖ *Carbohydrates: 32g*
- ❖ *Protein: 6g*
- ❖ *Fat: 17g*
- ❖ *Fiber: 12g*

Chia Seed Pudding with Berries

INGREDIENTS

1. 1/4 cup chia seeds
2. 1 cup almond milk
3. 1 teaspoon vanilla extract
4. Mixed berries (strawberries, blueberries)

INSTRUCTIONS

1. 1/4 cup chia seeds
2. 1 cup almond milk
3. 1 teaspoon vanilla extract
4. Mixed berries (strawberries, blueberries)
5. Instructions:
6. Mix chia seeds, almond milk, and vanilla extract in a bowl.
7. Refrigerate for a few hours or overnight until thickened.
8. Serve with mixed berries on top.

NUTRITION PER SERVING

- ❖ *Calories: 180*
- ❖ *Carbohydrates: 18g*
- ❖ *Protein: 5g*
- ❖ *Fat: 10g*
- ❖ *Fiber: 12g*

Avocado Toast with Tomato

INGREDIENTS

1. 2 slices whole grain bread
2. 1 ripe avocado
3. Sliced tomatoes
4. Lemon juice
5. Salt and pepper

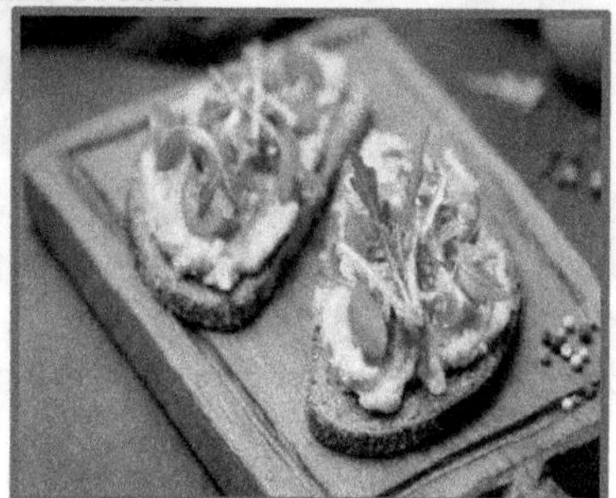

INSTRUCTIONS

1. Mash avocado, spread it on toasted bread.
2. Top with sliced tomatoes, a squeeze of lemon juice, salt, and pepper.

NUTRITION PER SERVING

- ❖ *Calories: 250*
- ❖ *Carbohydrates: 30g*
- ❖ *Protein: 7g*
- ❖ *Fat: 12g*
- ❖ *Fiber: 10g*

Quinoa Breakfast Bowl

INGREDIENTS

1. 1 cup cooked quinoa
2. 1/2 cup mixed berries
3. 1 tablespoon almond butter
4. 1 teaspoon honey

INSTRUCTIONS

1. Place cooked quinoa in a bowl.
2. Top with mixed berries, almond butter, and a drizzle of honey.

NUTRITION PER SERVING

- ❖ *Calories: 320*
- ❖ *Carbohydrates: 50g*
- ❖ *Protein: 9g*
- ❖ *Fat: 9g*
- ❖ *Fiber: 8g*

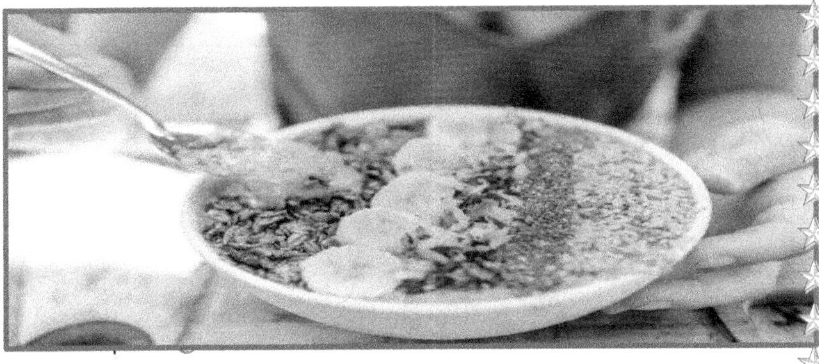

Almond Flour Pancakes

INGREDIENTS

1. 1 cup almond flour
2. 2 eggs
3. 1/2 teaspoon baking powder
4. 1 tablespoon coconut oil (for cooking)

INSTRUCTIONS

1. Mix almond flour, eggs, and baking powder in a bowl.
2. Heat coconut oil in a pan, pour batter, cook until golden.

NUTRITION PER SERVING

- ❖ *Calories: 280*
- ❖ *Carbohydrates: 8g*
- ❖ *Protein: 12g*
- ❖ *Fat: 24g*
- ❖ *Fiber: 4g*

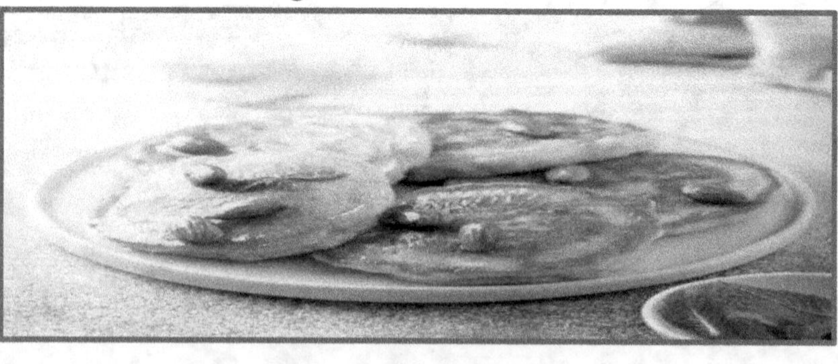

Spinach and Mushroom Omelette

INGREDIENTS

1. 2 eggs
2. Handful of spinach
3. Sliced mushrooms
4. 1 tablespoon olive oil

INSTRUCTIONS

1. Whisk eggs, pour into a heated pan with olive oil.
2. Add spinach and mushrooms, fold when cooked through.

NUTRITION PER SERVING

- *Calories: 210*
- *Carbohydrates: 3g*
- *Protein: 13g*
- *Fat: 16g*
- *Fiber: 2g*

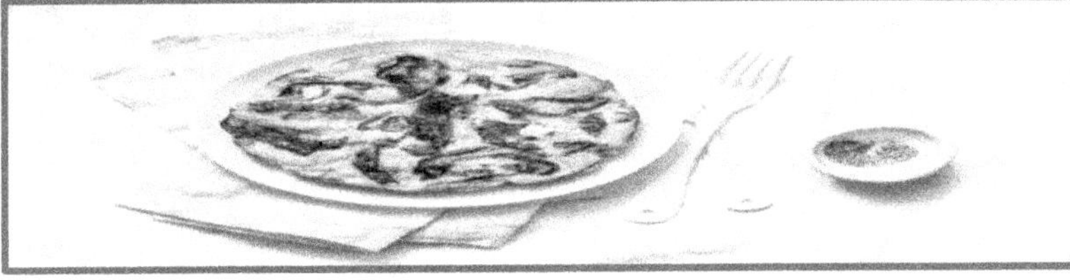

Coconut Yogurt Parfait

INGREDIENTS

1. 1 cup coconut yogurt
2. 1/4 cup granola
3. Sliced kiwi and pineapple

INSTRUCTIONS

Layer coconut yogurt, granola, and fruit in a glass. Repeat layers, ending with fruit on top.

NUTRITION PER SERVING

- ❖ *Calories: 280*
- ❖ *Carbohydrates: 40g*
- ❖ *Protein: 4g*
- ❖ *Fat: 12g*
- ❖ *Fiber: 6g*

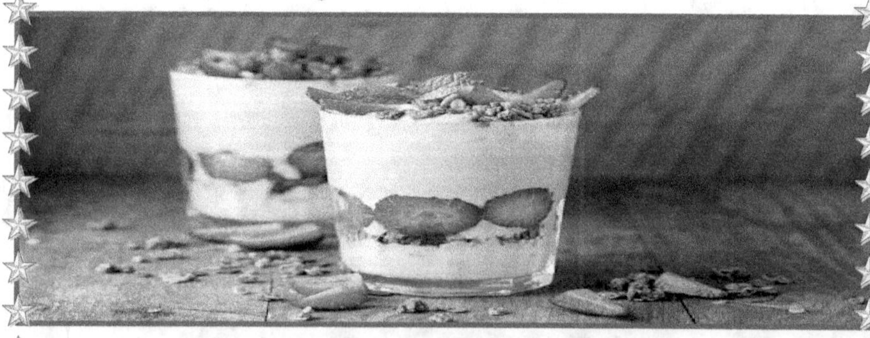

Berry and Spinach Smoothie

INGREDIENTS

1. 1 cup mixed berries
2. Handful of spinach
3. 1/2 cup coconut water
4. 1 tablespoon hemp seeds

INSTRUCTIONS

1. Blend berries, spinach, and coconut water until smooth.
2. Add hemp seeds and blend for a few seconds.

NUTRITION PER SERVING

- ❖ *Calories: 200*
- ❖ *Carbohydrates: 25g*
- ❖ *Protein: 6g*
- ❖ *Fat: 8g*
- ❖ *Fiber: 9g*

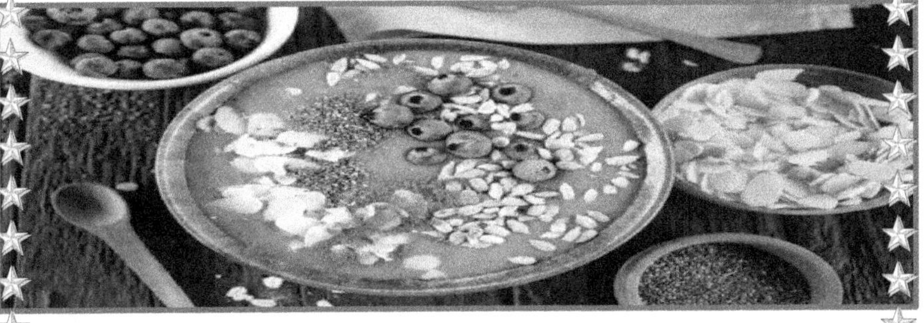

Buckwheat Porridge with Almonds

INGREDIENTS

1. 1/2 cup buckwheat groats
2. 1 cup almond milk
3. Sliced almonds
4. Cinnamon and honey (optional)

INSTRUCTIONS

1. Cook buckwheat groats in almond milk until soft.
2. Serve topped with sliced almonds and a sprinkle of cinnamon.

NUTRITION PER SERVING

- ❖ *Calories: 260*
- ❖ *Carbohydrates: 35g*
- ❖ *Protein: 9g*
- ❖ *Fat: 10g*
- ❖ *Fiber: 6g*

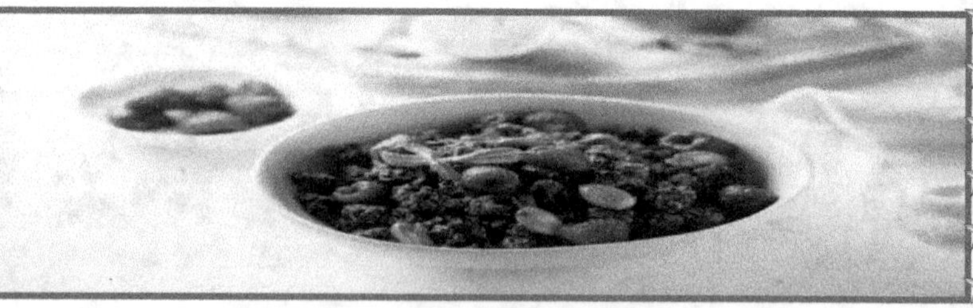

Tofu Scramble with Veggies

INGREDIENTS

1. 1/2 block tofu
2. Sliced bell peppers, onions, and tomatoes
3. 1 tablespoon olive oil
4. Turmeric, cumin, and paprika (for seasoning)

INSTRUCTIONS

Crumble tofu in a pan with olive oil and spices.
Add sliced veggies, cook until tender.

NUTRITION PER SERVING

- ❖ *Calories: 240*
- ❖ *Carbohydrates: 12g*
- ❖ *Protein: 15g*
- ❖ *Fat: 14g*
- ❖ *Fiber: 5g*

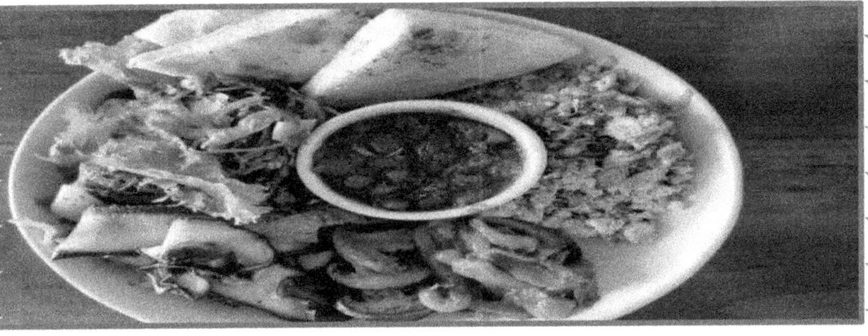

Alkaline Lunch Recipes for Cancer Defense

Alkaline Veggie Stir-Fry

INGREDIENTS

1. 2 cups mixed vegetables (bell peppers, broccoli, carrots)
2. 1 tablespoon coconut oil
3. 2 cloves garlic (minced)
4. 1-inch piece of ginger (grated)
5. 2 tablespoons tamari sauce (low sodium)
6. 1 cup quinoa (cooked)

INSTRUCTIONS

1. Heat coconut oil in a pan, add minced garlic and grated ginger.
2. Stir in mixed vegetables and sauté until tender.
3. Add tamari sauce and cooked quinoa, stir until well combined.
4. Serve hot.

NUTRITION PER SERVING

- ❖ *Calories: 280*
- ❖ *Carbohydrates: 45g*
- ❖ *Protein: 10g*
- ❖ *Fat: 7g*

Lemon-Herb Baked Salmon

INGREDIENTS

1. 4 salmon fillets
2. 2 tablespoons olive oil
3. Juice of 1 lemon
4. 2 teaspoons chopped fresh herbs (parsley, thyme)
5. Salt and pepper to taste

INSTRUCTIONS

1. Preheat oven to 375°F (190°C).
2. Place salmon fillets on a baking sheet.
3. Mix olive oil, lemon juice, herbs, salt, and pepper, then brush over the salmon.
4. Bake for 15-20 minutes until salmon is cooked through.
5. Serve with a side of steamed vegetables.

NUTRITION PER SERVING

- ❖ *Calories: 280*
- ❖ *Carbohydrates: 0g*
- ❖ *Protein: 25g*
- ❖ *Fat: 18g*

Chickpea Spinach Salad

INGREDIENTS

1. 1 can chickpeas (drained and rinsed)
2. 2 cups fresh spinach
3. 1 cucumber (sliced)
4. 1 bell pepper (sliced)
5. 2 tablespoons balsamic vinegar
6. 1 tablespoon olive oil

INSTRUCTIONS

1. Mix chickpeas, spinach, cucumber, and bell pepper in a bowl.
2. Drizzle with balsamic vinegar and olive oil, toss to coat.
3. Serve chilled.

NUTRITION PER SERVING

- ❖ *Calories: 220*
- ❖ *Carbohydrates: 32g*
- ❖ *Protein: 8g*
- ❖ *Fat: 8g*

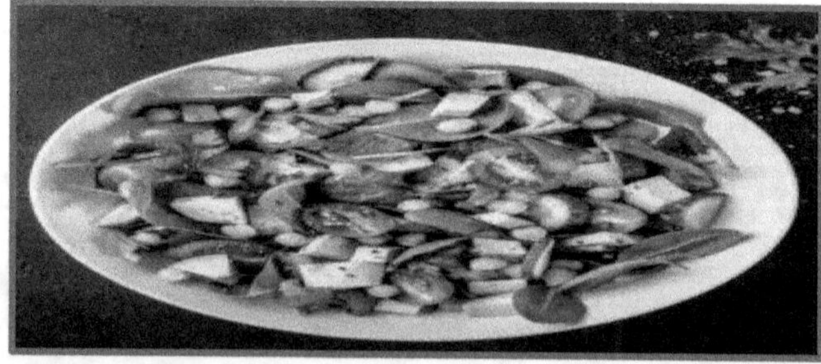

Quinoa Stuffed Bell Peppers

INGREDIENTS

1. 4 bell peppers (halved and deseeded)
2. 1 cup quinoa (cooked)
3. 1 can black beans (drained and rinsed)
4. 1 cup diced tomatoes
5. 1 teaspoon cumin
6. 1 teaspoon paprika
7. Salt and pepper to taste

INSTRUCTIONS

1. Preheat oven to 375°F (190°C).
2. In a bowl, mix cooked quinoa, black beans, diced tomatoes, cumin, paprika, salt, and pepper.
3. Stuff the halved bell peppers with the quinoa mixture.
4. Bake for 25-30 minutes until peppers are tender.
5. Serve hot.

NUTRITION PER SERVING

- ❖ *Calories: 240*
- ❖ *Carbohydrates: 45g*
- ❖ *Protein: 10g*
- ❖ *Fat: 3g*

Tofu Veggie Stir-Fry

INGREDIENTS

1. 1 block tofu (pressed and cubed)
2. 2 cups mixed vegetables (broccoli, bell peppers, snap peas)
3. 2 tablespoons sesame oil
4. 3 tablespoons low-sodium soy sauce
5. 1 tablespoon rice vinegar
6. 1 teaspoon minced garlic
7. 1 teaspoon grated ginger

INSTRUCTIONS

1. Heat sesame oil in a pan, add tofu cubes and stir-fry until golden.
2. Add mixed vegetables, garlic, and ginger, sauté until veggies are tender.
3. Pour in soy sauce and rice vinegar, toss until well coated.
4. Serve with brown rice or quinoa.

NUTRITION PER SERVING

- ❖ *Calories: 280*
- ❖ *Carbohydrates: 18g*
- ❖ *Protein: 20g*
- ❖ *Fat: 15g*

Lentil Vegetable Soup

INGREDIENTS

1. 1 cup lentils (rinsed)
2. 4 cups vegetable broth
3. 2 carrots (diced)
4. 2 celery stalks (chopped)
5. 1 onion (chopped)
6. 2 cloves garlic (minced)
7. 1 teaspoon turmeric
8. 1 teaspoon dried thyme
9. Salt and pepper to taste

INSTRUCTIONS

1. In a pot, sauté onions, garlic, carrots, and celery until softened.
2. Add lentils, vegetable broth, turmeric, thyme, salt, and pepper.
3. Simmer for 25-30 minutes until lentils are tender.
4. Serve hot as a nourishing soup.

NUTRITION PER SERVING

- ❖ *Calories: 220*
- ❖ *Carbohydrates: 38g*
- ❖ *Protein: 15g*
- ❖ *Fat: 1g*

Spinach and Chickpea Curry

INGREDIENTS

1. 2 cups cooked chickpeas
2. 2 cups fresh spinach
3. 1 onion (chopped)
4. 2 tomatoes (diced)
5. 2 cloves garlic (minced)
6. 1-inch piece of ginger (grated)
7. 1 teaspoon turmeric
8. 1 teaspoon cumin
9. 1 teaspoon coriander
10. 1 tablespoon coconut oil
11. Salt and pepper to taste

INSTRUCTIONS

1. Heat coconut oil in a pan, sauté onions, garlic, and ginger until fragrant.
2. Add diced tomatoes and cook until softened.
3. Stir in turmeric, cumin, coriander, salt, and pepper.
4. Add chickpeas and simmer for 10 minutes.
5. Add spinach, cover, and cook until wilted.
6. Serve with brown rice or quinoa.

NUTRITION PER SERVING

- *Calories: 280*
- *Carbohydrates: 40g*
- *Protein: 14g*
- *Fat: 8g*

Mediterranean Quinoa Salad

INGREDIENTS

1. 2 cups cooked quinoa
2. 1 cucumber (diced)
3. 1 bell pepper (chopped)
4. ½ red onion (sliced)
5. ½ cup cherry tomatoes (halved)
6. ¼ cup Kalamata olives (pitted)
7. 2 tablespoons olive oil
8. Juice of 1 lemon
9. 2 tablespoons chopped fresh parsley
10. Salt and pepper to taste

INSTRUCTIONS

1. In a bowl, mix quinoa, cucumber, bell pepper, red onion, cherry tomatoes, and olives.
2. Drizzle with olive oil and lemon juice, toss to combine.
3. Season with salt, pepper, and garnish with chopped parsley.
4. Serve chilled.

NUTRITION PER SERVING

- ❖ *Calories: 260*
- ❖ *Carbohydrates: 35g*
- ❖ *Protein: 6g*
- ❖ *Fat: 10g*

Baked Eggplant and Tomato Casserole

INGREDIENTS

1. 2 eggplants (sliced)
2. 4 tomatoes (sliced)
3. 2 cloves garlic (minced)
4. ½ cup breadcrumbs (whole grain)
5. 2 tablespoons olive oil
6. 2 tablespoons chopped fresh basil
7. Salt and pepper to taste

INSTRUCTIONS

1. Preheat oven to 375°F (190°C).
2. Arrange alternating slices of eggplant and tomato in a baking dish.
3. Mix minced garlic, breadcrumbs, olive oil, basil, salt, and pepper.
4. Spread breadcrumb mixture over the eggplant and tomato.
5. Bake for 30-35 minutes until golden brown.
6. Serve warm.

NUTRITION PER SERVING

- *Calories: 210*
- *Carbohydrates: 30g*
- *Protein: 6g*
- *Fat: 8g*

Tofu and Vegetable Brown Rice Bowl

INGREDIENTS

1. 1 block tofu (pressed and cubed)
2. 2 cups mixed vegetables (bell peppers, broccoli, carrots)
3. 2 cups cooked brown rice
4. 2 tablespoons low-sodium soy sauce
5. 1 tablespoon rice vinegar
6. 1 tablespoon sesame seeds
7. 1 tablespoon chopped green onions

INSTRUCTIONS

1. Sauté tofu cubes until golden brown.
2. Add mixed vegetables and stir-fry until tender.
3. Mix in cooked brown rice, soy sauce, and rice vinegar.
4. Top with sesame seeds and green onions.
5. Serve hot.

NUTRITION PER SERVING

- *Calories: 290*
- *Carbohydrates: 40g*
- *Protein: 16g*
- *Fat: 9g*

Alkaline Snacks Recipes for Cancer Defense

Alkaline Veggie Sticks with Hummus

INGREDIENTS

1. Carrot sticks
2. Celery sticks
3. Cucumber slices
4. Homemade hummus (chickpeas, tahini, lemon juice, garlic, olive oil, salt)

INSTRUCTIONS

1. Wash and cut vegetables into sticks or slices.
2. Prepare hummus by blending chickpeas, tahini, lemon juice, garlic, and olive oil until smooth.
3. Serve veggie sticks with homemade hummus.

NUTRITION PER SERVING

- *Calories: 120*
- *Protein: 5g*
- *Carbohydrates: 15g*
- *Fiber: 6g*
- *Fat: 6g*

Chia Seed Pudding with Berries

INGREDIENTS

1. 2 tablespoons chia seeds
2. 1 cup almond milk
3. ½ teaspoon vanilla extract
4. Mixed berries (strawberries, blueberries, raspberries)

INSTRUCTIONS

1. Mix chia seeds, almond milk, and vanilla extract in a bowl.
2. Refrigerate for at least 2 hours or overnight until the mixture thickens.
3. Top with mixed berries before serving.

NUTRITION PER SERVING

- ❖ *Calories: 150*
- ❖ *Protein: 5g*
- ❖ *Carbohydrates: 20g*
- ❖ *Fiber: 10g*
- ❖ *Fat: 7g*

Almond Butter on Rice Cakes

INGREDIENTS

1. Rice cakes
2. Almond butter (unsweetened)

INSTRUCTIONS

1. Spread almond butter generously on rice cakes.
2. Serve as a quick, crunchy snack.

NUTRITION PER SERVING

- ❖ *Calories: 100*
- ❖ *Protein: 4g*
- ❖ *Carbohydrates: 12g*
- ❖ *Fiber: 2g*
- ❖ *Fat: 5g*

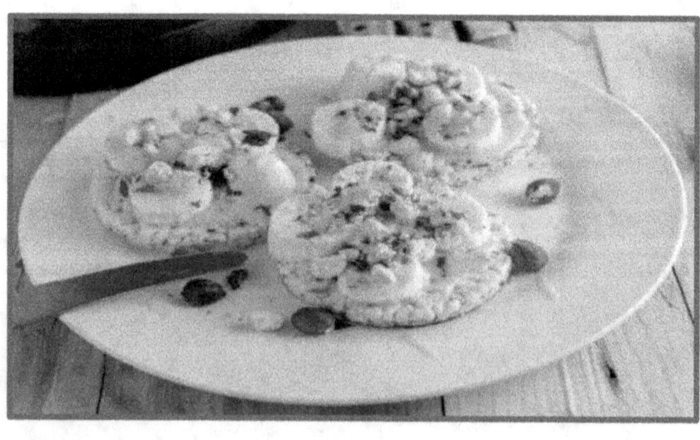

Guacamole with Veggie Chips

INGREDIENTS

1. Ripe avocados
2. Diced tomatoes
3. Chopped cilantro
4. Lime juice
5. Salt
6. Veggie chips (baked beet, sweet potato, or kale chips)

INSTRUCTIONS

1. Mash avocados and mix with diced tomatoes, cilantro, lime juice, and salt.
2. Serve with veggie chips for dipping.

NUTRITION PER SERVING

- ❖ *Calories: 130*
- ❖ *Protein: 2g*
- ❖ *Carbohydrates: 8g*
- ❖ *Fiber: 6g*
- ❖ *Fat: 10g*

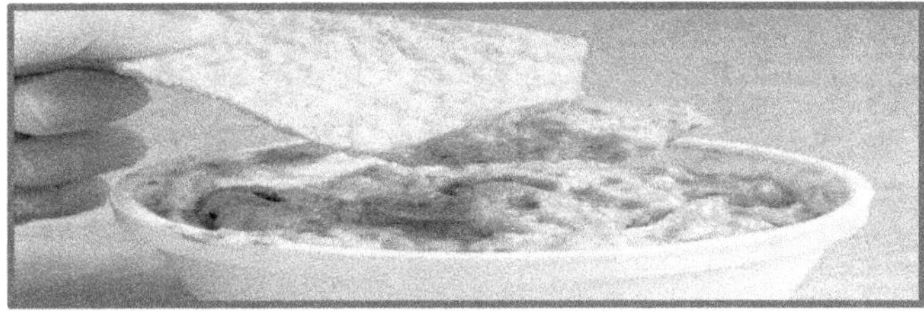

Raw Nuts and Seeds Mix

INGREDIENTS

1. Almonds
2. Walnuts
3. Pumpkin seeds
4. Sunflower seeds

INSTRUCTIONS

1. Mix equal parts of almonds, walnuts, pumpkin seeds, and sunflower seeds.
2. Portion into small servings for a quick, nutrient-dense snack.

NUTRITION PER SERVING

- *Calories: 180*
- *Protein: 7g*
- *Carbohydrates: 5g*
- *Fiber: 4g*
- *Fat: 15g*

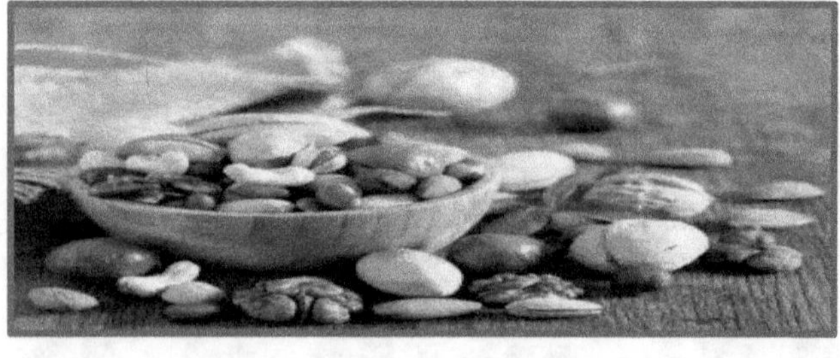

Baked Kale Chips

INGREDIENTS

1. Fresh kale leaves
2. Olive oil
3. Sea salt

INSTRUCTIONS

1. Remove stems from kale and tear leaves into bite-sized pieces.
2. Toss kale with olive oil and a pinch of sea salt.
3. Bake at 350°F (175°C) for 10-15 minutes until crispy.

NUTRITION PER SERVING

- ❖ *Calories: 50*
- ❖ *Protein: 3g*
- ❖ *Carbohydrates: 8g*
- ❖ *Fiber: 2g*
- ❖ *Fat: 2g*

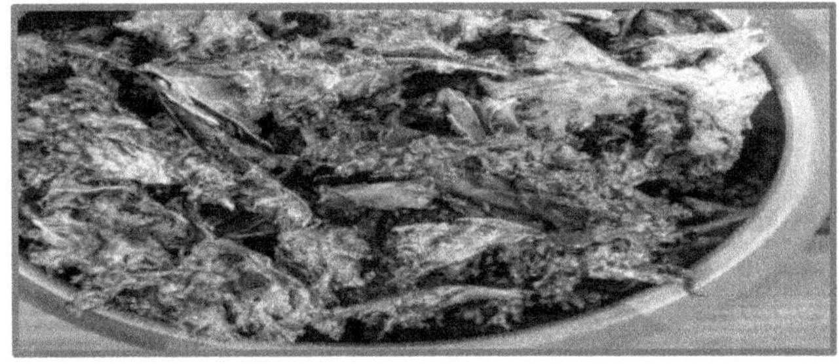

Apple Slices with Almond Butter

INGREDIENTS

1. Apples (sliced)
2. Almond butter (unsweetened)

INSTRUCTIONS

1. Spread almond butter on apple slices.
2. Enjoy this simple yet satisfying snack option.

NUTRITION PER SERVING

- ❖ *Calories: 120*
- ❖ *Protein: 3g*
- ❖ *Carbohydrates: 18g*
- ❖ *Fiber: 5g*
- ❖ *Fat: 6g*

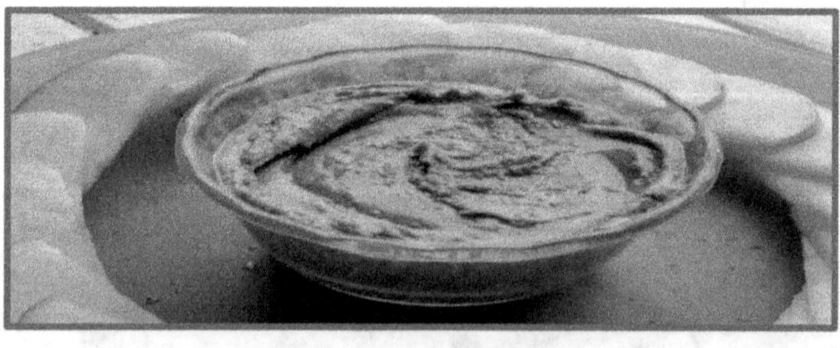

Hummus Stuffed Bell Peppers

INGREDIENTS

1. Mini bell peppers
2. Homemade hummus

INSTRUCTIONS

1. Cut mini bell peppers in half lengthwise and remove seeds.
2. Stuff each half with homemade hummus.

NUTRITION PER SERVING

- ❖ *Calories: 70*
- ❖ *Protein: 3g*
- ❖ *Carbohydrates: 9g*
- ❖ *Fiber: 3g*
- ❖ *Fat: 3g*

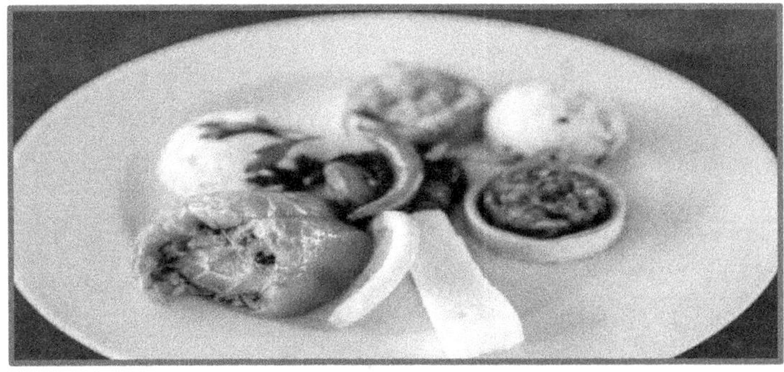

Cucumber Slices with Greek Yogurt Dip

INGREDIENTS

1. Cucumber (sliced)
2. Greek yogurt (unsweetened)
3. Fresh dill (chopped)
4. Lemon juice
5. Salt

INSTRUCTIONS

1. Mix Greek yogurt with chopped dill, lemon juice, and a pinch of salt.
2. Use as a dip for cucumber slices.

NUTRITION PER SERVING

- *Calories: 60*
- *Protein: 4g*
- *Carbohydrates: 7g*
- *Fiber: 1g*
- *Fat: 2g*

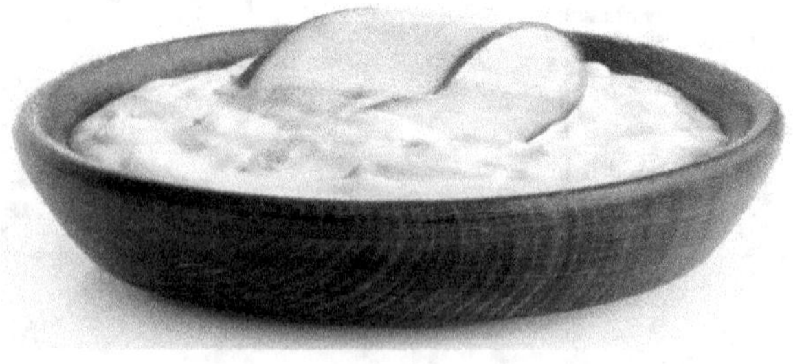

Berry Smoothie Bowl

INGREDIENTS

1. Mixed berries (frozen or fresh)
2. Almond milk
3. Chia seeds
4. Banana (optional for added sweetness)

INSTRUCTIONS

1. Blend mixed berries, almond milk, and chia seeds until smooth.
2. Pour into a bowl and top with additional berries or sliced fruits.

NUTRITION PER SERVING

- ❖ *Calories: 140*
- ❖ *Protein: 3g*
- ❖ *Carbohydrates: 20g*
- ❖ *Fiber: 8g*
- ❖ *Fat: 5g*

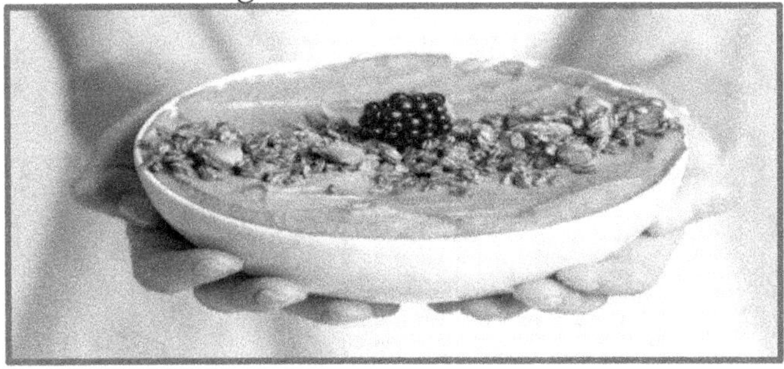

Alkaline Dinner Recipes for Cancer Defense

Lemon Herb Baked Chicken

INGREDIENTS

1. 4 boneless chicken breasts
2. 2 tablespoons olive oil
3. Juice of 1 lemon
4. 3 cloves garlic, minced
5. Herbs (rosemary, thyme)

INSTRUCTIONS

1. Preheat oven to 375°F (190°C).
2. Mix olive oil, lemon juice, minced garlic, and herbs.
3. Coat chicken breasts with the mixture and bake for 25-30 mins.

NUTRITION PER SERVING

- ❖ *Calories: 250*
- ❖ *Protein: 30g*
- ❖ *Fat: 12g*
- ❖ *Carbs: 3g*

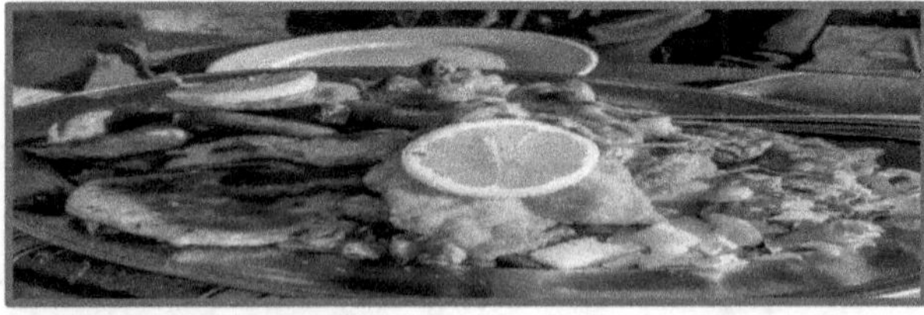

Quinoa-Stuffed Bell Peppers

INGREDIENTS

1. 1 cup quinoa
2. 4 bell peppers
3. 1 can black beans
4. Diced veggies (tomatoes, onions, corn)
5. Spices (cumin, paprika)

INSTRUCTIONS

1. Cook quinoa according to package instructions.
2. Mix cooked quinoa, black beans, diced veggies, and spices.
3. Stuff bell peppers and bake for 25-30 mins.

NUTRITION PER SERVING

- ❖ *Calories: 280*
- ❖ *Protein: 10g*
- ❖ *Fat: 2g*
- ❖ *Carbs: 50g*

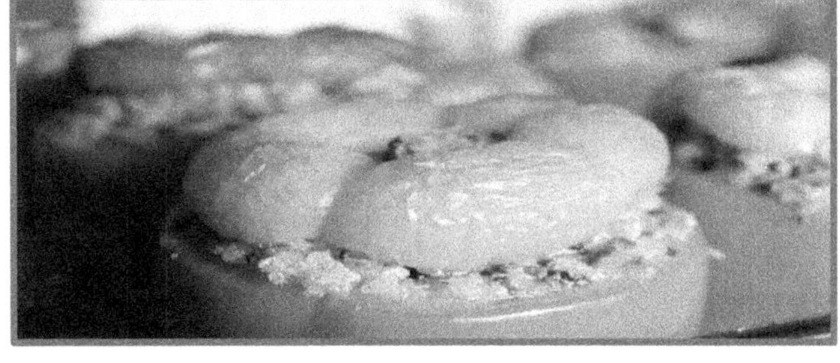

Seared Tofu with Steamed Broccoli

INGREDIENTS

1. 1 block tofu
2. Soy sauce
3. Fresh ginger
4. Broccoli

INSTRUCTIONS

1. Press tofu to remove excess moisture and slice.
2. Sear tofu in a pan and season with soy sauce and ginger.
3. Steam broccoli until tender-crisp.

NUTRITION PER SERVING

- ❖ *Calories: 180*
- ❖ *Protein: 15g*
- ❖ *Fat: 8g*
- ❖ *Carbs: 14g*

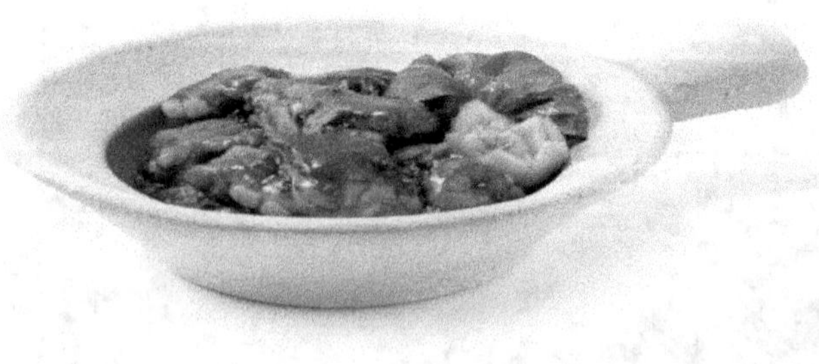

Lemon-Garlic Baked Salmon

INGREDIENTS

1. 4 salmon fillets
2. 2 tablespoons olive oil
3. Zest of 1 lemon
4. 2 cloves garlic, minced
5. Seasoning (dill, paprika)

INSTRUCTIONS

1. Preheat oven to 400°F (200°C).
2. Mix olive oil, lemon zest, minced garlic, and seasoning.
3. Coat salmon fillets, bake for 12-15 mins.

NUTRITION PER SERVING

- ❖ *Calories: 280*
- ❖ *Protein: 25g*
- ❖ *Fat: 18g*
- ❖ *Carbs: 1g*

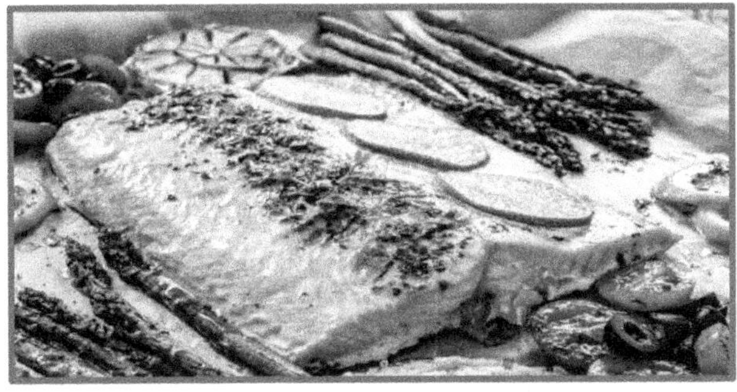

Vegetable Stir-Fry with Quinoa

INGREDIENTS

1. Assorted veggies
2. Quinoa
3. Tofu or edamame
4. Sesame oil, soy sauce

INSTRUCTIONS

1. Sauté diced veggies (bell peppers, broccoli, carrots) in sesame oil.
2. Add tofu or edamame, soy sauce, and spices.
3. Serve over cooked quinoa.

NUTRITION PER SERVING

- ❖ *Calories: 220*
- ❖ *Protein: 10g*
- ❖ *Fat: 6g*
- ❖ *Carbs: 35g*

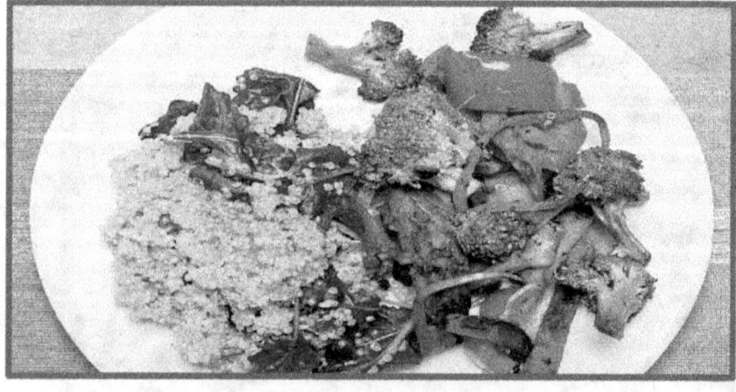

Lentil Curry with Brown Rice

INGREDIENTS

1. 2 cups lentils
2. Coconut milk
3. Brown rice
4. Curry spices, onions, garlic

INSTRUCTIONS

1. Sauté onions, garlic, and spices in a pot.
2. Add lentils, coconut milk, and simmer until cooked.
3. Serve over brown rice.

NUTRITION PER SERVING

- ❖ *Calories: 320*
- ❖ *Protein: 18g*
- ❖ *Fat: 6g*
- ❖ *Carbs: 50g*

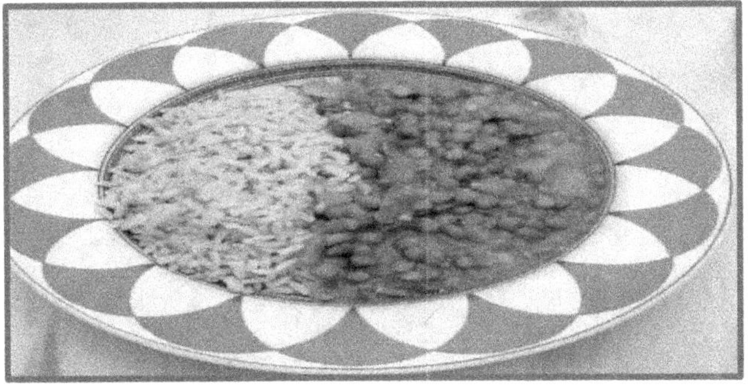

Baked Eggplant Parmesan

INGREDIENTS

1. 2 eggplants
2. Eggs, breadcrumbs
3. Marinara sauce, mozzarella cheese

INSTRUCTIONS

1. Slice eggplant, dip in egg, coat with breadcrumbs.
2. Bake until golden, layer with marinara sauce and cheese.
3. Bake until cheese melts and bubbles.

NUTRITION PER SERVING

- ❖ *Calories: 260*
- ❖ *Protein: 10g*
- ❖ *Fat: 10g*
- ❖ *Carbs: 35g*

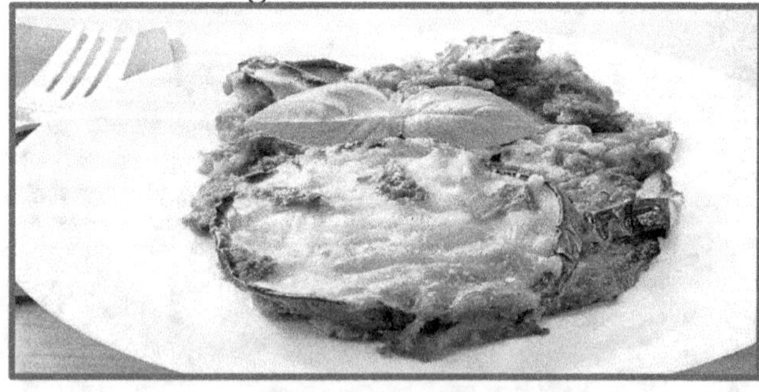

Lemon-Garlic Shrimp Stir-Fry

INGREDIENTS

1. Shrimp
2. Assorted veggies
3. Lemon juice, soy sauce
4. Red pepper flakes
5.

INSTRUCTIONS

1. Sauté shrimp, garlic, and veggies in olive oil.
2. Add lemon juice, soy sauce, and red pepper flakes.
3. Serve over quinoa or brown rice.

NUTRITION PER SERVING

❖ *Calories: 220*
❖ *Protein: 25g*
❖ *Fat: 6g*
❖ *Carbs: 18g*

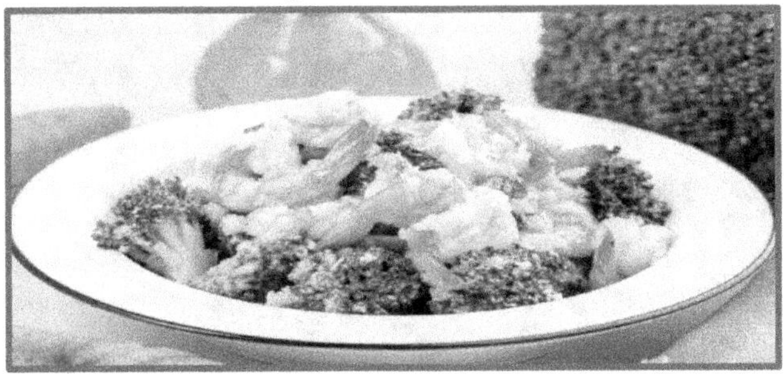

Spinach and Chickpea Curry

INGREDIENTS

1. Chickpeas
2. Spinach
3. Coconut milk
4. Quinoa or brown rice

INSTRUCTIONS

1. Sauté onions, garlic, and curry spices in a pan.
2. Add chickpeas, spinach, coconut milk, and simmer.
3. Serve over quinoa or brown rice.

NUTRITION PER SERVING

- ❖ *Calories: 280*
- ❖ *Protein: 12g*
- ❖ *Fat: 8g*
- ❖ *Carbs: 40g*

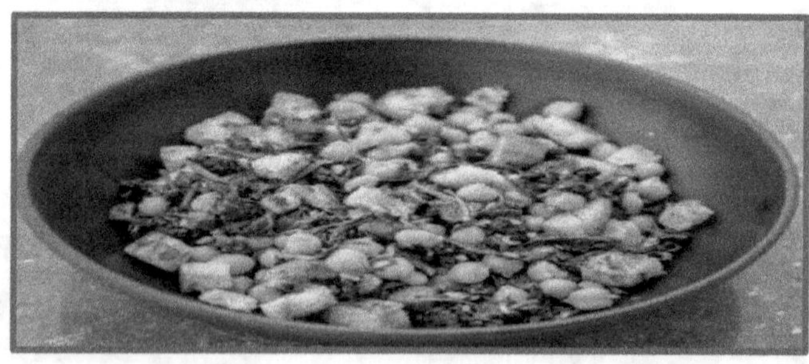

Grilled Portobello Mushrooms with Herbs

INGREDIENTS

1. Portobello mushrooms
2. Olive oil
3. Fresh herbs (rosemary, thyme)

INSTRUCTIONS

1. Marinate portobello mushrooms in olive oil and herbs.
2. Grill until tender and serve with a side salad.

NUTRITION PER SERVING

- ❖ *Calories: 90*
- ❖ *Protein: 5g*
- ❖ *Fat: 7g*
- ❖ *Carbs: 5g*

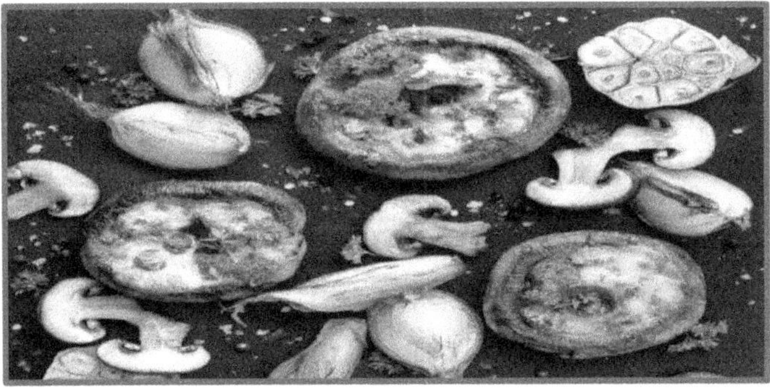

Alkaline Desserts Recipes for Cancer Defense

Berry Chia Seed Pudding

INGREDIENTS

1. ½ cup mixed berries (blueberries, strawberries)
2. 2 tablespoons chia seeds
3. 1 cup almond milk
4. ½ teaspoon vanilla extract

INSTRUCTIONS

1. Mix chia seeds, almond milk, and vanilla extract in a bowl.
2. Let it sit for 15 minutes, stirring occasionally.
3. Layer chia pudding with mixed berries.
4. Refrigerate for at least an hour before serving.

NUTRITION PER SERVING

- ❖ *Calories: 150*
- ❖ *Protein: 4g*
- ❖ *Carbohydrates: 18g*
- ❖ *Fiber: 9g*

Almond Butter Banana Bites

INGREDIENTS

1. 2 bananas, sliced
2. 4 tablespoons almond butter
3. 2 tablespoons shredded coconut (optional)

INSTRUCTIONS

1. Spread almond butter on banana slices.
2. Sprinkle shredded coconut on top (optional).
3. Freeze for 30 minutes before serving.

NUTRITION PER SERVING

- ❖ *Calories: 120*
- ❖ *Protein: 3g*
- ❖ *Carbohydrates: 15g*
- ❖ *Fat: 6g*

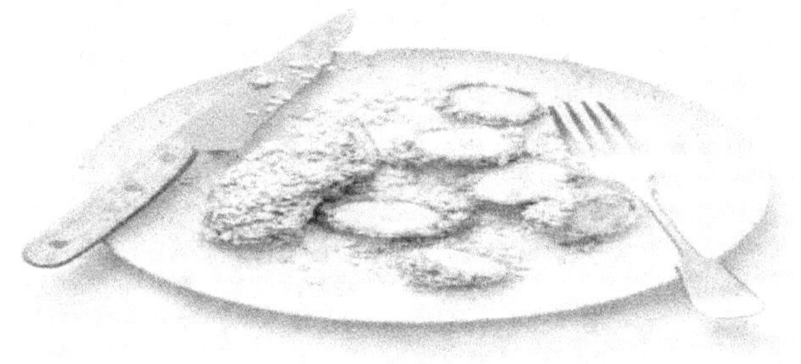

Citrus Fruit Salad

INGREDIENTS

1. 1 grapefruit, segmented
2. 2 oranges, segmented
3. 1 tablespoon honey (optional)
4. Fresh mint leaves for garnish

INSTRUCTIONS

1. Combine grapefruit and orange segments in a bowl.
2. Drizzle honey (optional) and garnish with mint leaves.

NUTRITION PER SERVING

- ❖ *Calories: 80*
- ❖ *Protein: 1g*
- ❖ *Carbohydrates: 20g*
- ❖ *Fiber: 4g*

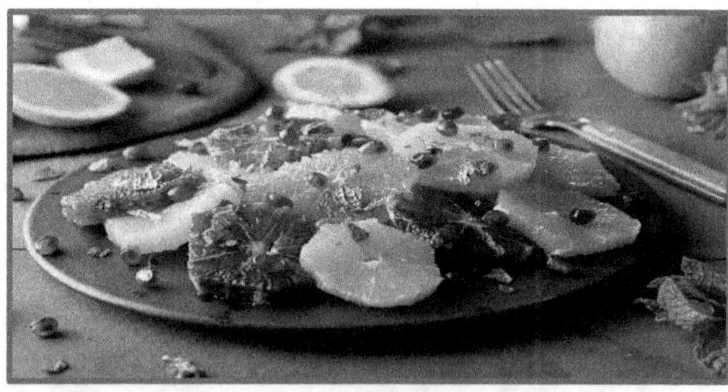

Coconut Yogurt Parfait

INGREDIENTS

1. 1 cup coconut yogurt
2. ½ cup mixed berries
3. 2 tablespoons granola

INSTRUCTIONS

1. Layer coconut yogurt, mixed berries, and granola in a glass.
2. Repeat layers as desired.
3. Serve chilled.

NUTRITION PER SERVING

❖ *Calories: 180*
❖ *Protein: 3g*
❖ *Carbohydrates: 25g*
❖ *Fat: 8g*

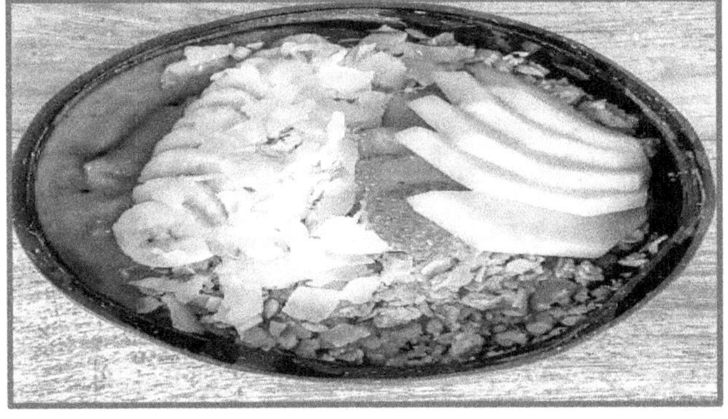

Avocado Chocolate Mousse

INGREDIENTS

1. 2 ripe avocados
2. ¼ cup cocoa powder
3. 3 tablespoons maple syrup
4. ½ teaspoon vanilla extract

INSTRUCTIONS

1. Blend avocados, cocoa powder, maple syrup, and vanilla until smooth.
2. Refrigerate for 30 minutes before serving.

NUTRITION PER SERVING

- ❖ *Calories: 200*
- ❖ *Protein: 3g*
- ❖ *Carbohydrates: 18g*
- ❖ *Fat: 15g*

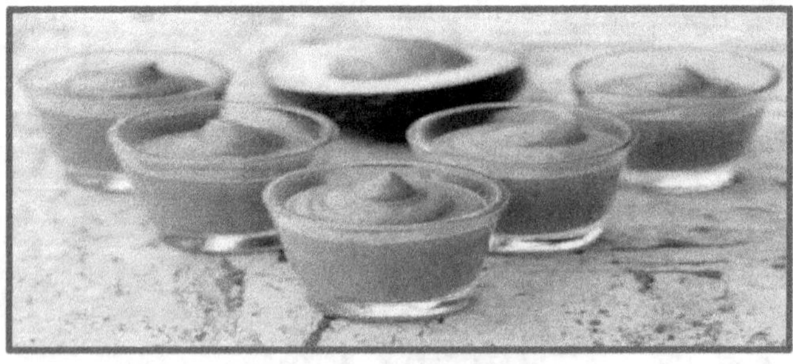

Pineapple Coconut Sorbet

INGREDIENTS

1. 2 cups frozen pineapple chunks
2. ½ cup coconut milk
3. 1 tablespoon honey (optional)

INSTRUCTIONS

1. Blend frozen pineapple, coconut milk, and honey until smooth.
2. Freeze for 2 hours before serving.

NUTRITION PER SERVING

- ❖ *Calories: 120*
- ❖ *Protein: 1g*
- ❖ *Carbohydrates: 30g*
- ❖ *Fat: 3g*

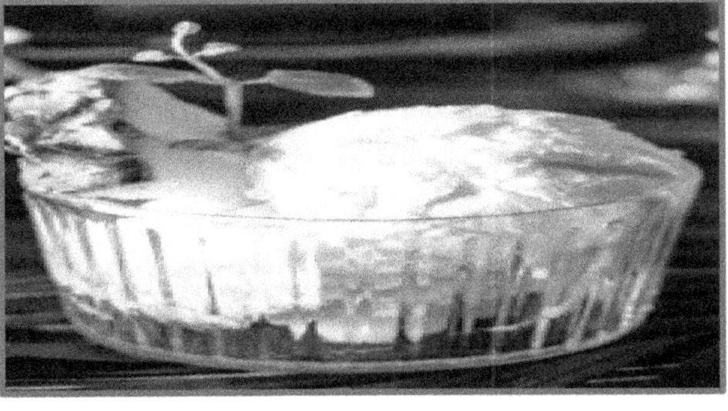

Alkaline Apple Crisp

INGREDIENTS

1. 4 apples, peeled and sliced
2. 1 cup oats
3. ½ cup almond flour
4. ¼ cup coconut oil
5. 2 tablespoons maple syrup

INSTRUCTIONS

1. Mix apples with maple syrup and place in a baking dish.
2. Combine oats, almond flour, and coconut oil. Sprinkle over apples.
3. Bake at 350°F for 30 minutes.

NUTRITION PER SERVING

- ❖ *Calories: 220*
- ❖ *Protein: 4g*
- ❖ *Carbohydrates: 35g*
- ❖ *Fat: 8g*

Lemon Ginger Turmeric Gummies

INGREDIENTS

1. 1 cup fresh lemon juice
2. 2 tablespoons honey
3. 2 teaspoons grated ginger
4. 1 teaspoon ground turmeric
5. 4 tablespoons gelatin powder

INSTRUCTIONS

1. Heat lemon juice, honey, ginger, and turmeric in a saucepan.
2. Whisk in gelatin until dissolved. Pour into molds.
3. Refrigerate for 2 hours before removing from molds.

NUTRITION PER SERVING

- *Calories: 30*
- *Protein: 3g*
- *Carbohydrates: 4g*
- *Fat: 0g*

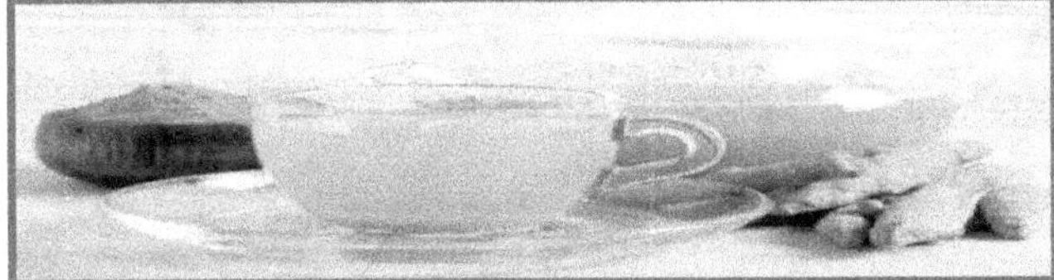

Watermelon Mint Popsicles

INGREDIENTS

1. 3 cups cubed watermelon
2. Juice of 1 lime
3. Fresh mint leaves

INSTRUCTIONS

1. Blend watermelon and lime juice until smooth.
2. Add fresh mint leaves and blend briefly.
3. Pour into popsicle molds and freeze.

NUTRITION PER SERVING

- ❖ *Calories: 40*
- ❖ *Protein: 1g*
- ❖ *Carbohydrates: 10g*
- ❖ *Fat: 0g*

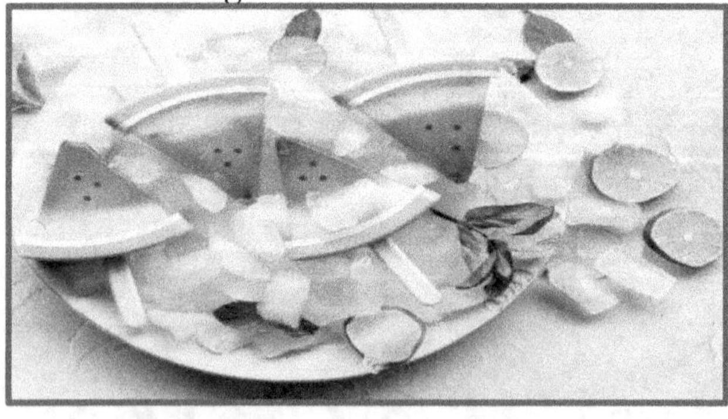

Blueberry Oatmeal Cookies

INGREDIENTS

1. 1 cup rolled oats
2. 1 ripe banana, mashed
3. ½ cup blueberries
4. 2 tablespoons maple syrup

INSTRUCTIONS

1. Mix oats, mashed banana, blueberries, and maple syrup.
2. Spoon onto a baking sheet and bake at 350°F for 15-20 minutes.

NUTRITION PER SERVING

- ❖ *Calories: 120*
- ❖ *Protein: 3g*
- ❖ *Carbohydrates: 25g*
- ❖ *Fat: 1g*

Alkaline Treats Recipes for Cancer Defense

Alkaline Berry Smoothie Bowl

INGREDIENTS

1. 1 cup mixed berries (strawberries, blueberries, raspberries)
2. 1 ripe banana
3. 1/2 cup spinach
4. 1/2 cup almond milk (unsweetened)
5. 1 tablespoon chia seeds

INSTRUCTIONS

1. Blend berries, banana, spinach, and almond milk until smooth.
2. Pour into a bowl and top with chia seeds.

NUTRITION PER SERVING

- ❖ *Calories: 180*
- ❖ *Carbohydrates: 35g*
- ❖ *Fiber: 9g*
- ❖ *Protein: 4g*
- ❖ *Fat: 5g*

Avocado Chocolate Mousse

INGREDIENTS

1. 2 ripe avocados
2. 1/4 cup raw cacao powder
3. 3 tablespoons maple syrup
4. 1 teaspoon vanilla extract

INSTRUCTIONS

1. Blend avocados, cacao powder, maple syrup, and vanilla extract until creamy.
2. Refrigerate for 1-2 hours before serving.

NUTRITION PER SERVING

- ❖ *Calories: 180*
- ❖ *Carbohydrates: 15g*
- ❖ *Fiber: 9g*
- ❖ *Protein: 3g*
- ❖ *Fat: 13g*

Alkaline Fruit Popsicles

INGREDIENTS

1. 1 cup mixed fruit (kiwi, pineapple, mango)
2. 2 cups coconut water
3. 1 tablespoon honey (optional)

INSTRUCTIONS

1. Slice fruits and place them into popsicle molds.
2. Pour coconut water over the fruit.
3. Freeze for at least 4 hours or until solid.

NUTRITION PER SERVING

- ❖ *Calories: 50*
- ❖ *Carbohydrates: 12g*
- ❖ *Fiber: 2g*
- ❖ *Protein: 1g*
- ❖ *Fat: 0g*

Coconut Chia Seed Pudding

INGREDIENTS

1. 1/4 cup chia seeds
2. 1 cup coconut milk
3. 1 tablespoon maple syrup
4. Fresh berries for topping

INSTRUCTIONS

1. Mix chia seeds, coconut milk, and maple syrup in a bowl.
2. Refrigerate for at least 4 hours or overnight.
3. Top with fresh berries before serving.

NUTRITION PER SERVING

- ❖ *Calories: 220*
- ❖ *Carbohydrates: 20g*
- ❖ *Fiber: 12g*
- ❖ *Protein: 4g*
- ❖ *Fat: 15g*

Almond Butter Energy Balls

INGREDIENTS

1. 1 cup rolled oats
2. 1/2 cup almond butter
3. 1/4 cup honey
4. 1/4 cup shredded coconut

INSTRUCTIONS

1. Mix oats, almond butter, honey, and shredded coconut in a bowl.
2. Roll into small balls and refrigerate for 30 minutes before serving.

NUTRITION PER SERVING

- ❖ *Calories: 120*
- ❖ *Carbohydrates: 15g*
- ❖ *Fiber: 2g*
- ❖ *Protein: 4g*
- ❖ *Fat: 6g*

Green Tea Matcha Nice Cream

INGREDIENTS

1. 3 ripe bananas (frozen)
2. 1 teaspoon matcha powder
3. 1/4 cup almond milk

INSTRUCTIONS

1. Blend frozen bananas, matcha powder, and almond milk until smooth.
2. Freeze for 1-2 hours for a firmer texture.

NUTRITION PER SERVING

- ❖ *Calories: 150*
- ❖ *Carbohydrates: 38g*
- ❖ *Fiber: 5g*
- ❖ *Protein: 2g*
- ❖ *Fat: 1g*

Baked Apples with Cinnamon

INGREDIENTS

1. 4 apples (cored)
2. 2 tablespoons maple syrup
3. 1 teaspoon cinnamon
4. Chopped nuts for topping (optional)

INSTRUCTIONS

1. Preheat oven to 350°F (175°C).
2. Mix maple syrup and cinnamon, then drizzle over cored apples.
3. Bake for 25-30 minutes until apples are tender.
4. Top with chopped nuts before serving.

NUTRITION PER SERVING

- ❖ *Calories: 120*
- ❖ *Carbohydrates: 30g*
- ❖ *Fiber: 6g*
- ❖ *Protein: 1g*
- ❖ *Fat: 0g*

Turmeric Golden Milk Latte

INGREDIENTS

1. 2 cups almond milk
2. 1 teaspoon turmeric
3. 1/2 teaspoon cinnamon
4. 1 tablespoon honey (optional)
5. Pinch of black pepper

INSTRUCTIONS

1. Warm almond milk in a saucepan.
2. Whisk in turmeric, cinnamon, honey, and black pepper until combined.
3. Pour into mugs and serve warm.

NUTRITION PER SERVING

- *Calories: 80*
- *Carbohydrates: 12g*
- *Fiber: 2g*
- *Protein: 1g*
- *Fat: 3g*

Spinach and Pineapple Sorbet

INGREDIENTS

1. 2 cups spinach
2. 2 cups frozen pineapple chunks
3. 1/2 cup coconut water
4. 1 tablespoon lime juice

INSTRUCTIONS

1. Blend spinach, frozen pineapple, coconut water, and lime juice until smooth.
2. Freeze for 1-2 hours for a sorbet-like consistency.

NUTRITION PER SERVING

- *Calories: 100*
- *Carbohydrates: 25g*
- *Fiber: 4g*
- *Protein: 2g*
- *Fat: 1g*

Alkaline Lemon Coconut Bars

INGREDIENTS

1. 1 cup shredded coconut
2. 1/4 cup coconut oil (melted)
3. 1/4 cup maple syrup
4. Zest of 1 lemon

INSTRUCTIONS

1. Mix shredded coconut, melted coconut oil, maple syrup, and lemon zest in a bowl.
2. Press mixture into a lined baking pan and freeze for 1 hour.
3. Cut into bars before serving.

NUTRITION PER SERVING

- ❖ *Calories: 120*
- ❖ *Carbohydrates: 10g*
- ❖ *Fiber: 2g*
- ❖ *Protein: 1g*
- ❖ *Fat: 9g*

Chapter 4

LIFESTYLE AND ADDITIONAL TIPS

Complementary Lifestyle Changes

1. Exercise regularly

Exercise Routine: Start a regular fitness regimen, such as jogging, yoga, weightlifting, or walking. Aim for at least 30 minutes of moderate exercise most days of the week.

Benefits: Exercise improves mood, improves circulation, boosts overall health, and may amplify the positive effects of an alkaline diet on well-being.

2. Decrease in Stress

Engage in stress-relieving activities such as deep breathing, mindfulness exercises, or meditation as part of your mindfulness practice.

Benefits: Reducing stress may improve overall health and strengthen the benefits of an alkaline diet that increases immunity and reduces inflammation.

3. Sound Sleep

Create a Sleep Schedule: Ensure that you receive enough sleep by creating a calming nightly routine, adhering to a regular sleep schedule, and ensuring sure your sleeping area is comfortable.

Benefits: Sleeping adequate sleep supports the body's natural healing processes, cellular regeneration, and overall health.

4. Routines for Drinking

Sufficient Water Intake: Drink water throughout the day to ensure that you are well hydrated. Try adding lemon to your beverage or utilizing alkaline water for potential alkalizing benefits.

The benefits of drinking adequate water include promoting bodily functions, aiding in digestion, flushing the body of impurities, and maintaining overall health.

5. Mindful Eating

Chew food thoroughly: Chew food thoroughly and slowly to enhance digestion and nutritional absorption. This is a method of mindful eating.

Include a variety of nutrient-dense, alkaline-producing items in your diet to keep it balanced, but also be mindful of portion sizes.

6. Diminishing Contaminants

Minimize Toxin Exposure: To help lessen your exposure to environmental toxins, pick organic food wherever possible, use natural cleaning products, and pay attention to the ingredients in personal care products.

Benefits: Reducing exposure to toxins improves overall health and may aid in achieving the goal of the alkaline diet, which is to reduce the body's toxic burden.

7. Social Connections

Nurture Relationships: Try to maintain strong ties with friends, family, and neighborhood associations by keeping in contact with individuals.

Benefits: Having close relationships with others fosters emotional and mental fortitude, both of which are advantageous to overall health.

8. Regular Medical Checkups

Frequent Health Assessments: Make an appointment for regular screenings and exams with medical professionals to guarantee early detection of any health concerns and preventive treatment.

Benefits: Routine physicals allow for the maintenance of optimal health and the prompt resolution of health issues.

9. Reducing Adverse Behaviors

Reducing or quitting smoking, excessive drinking, and processed meals high in sugar, fat, and artificial additives are some ways to avoid dangerous substances.

Benefits: Reducing unhealthy habits improves overall health and advances the alkaline diet's aim of promoting wellness.

10. Mind-Body Relationships

To enhance general well-being, consider mind-body practices that stress movement, breathing, and mindfulness, such as yoga, tai chi, or qigong.

Benefits: By reducing stress and improving flexibility, mind-body methods may improve overall health.

These complementary lifestyle changes, when combined with an alkaline diet, may have a synergistic effect that enhances overall health and may amp up the benefits of an alkaline-based dietary plan. It's crucial to tailor these lifestyle changes to the preferences of each individual and consult medical professionals for help on particular suggestions.

Exercise and Its Role in Cancer Prevention

Exercise is essential for preserving general health and has been linked to many advantages, such as a possible effect on cancer prevention. An outline of exercise's contribution to lowering the risk of cancer is provided below:

Exercise and the Prevention of Cancer

1. Diminishing Risk Elements

Weight management: By burning calories and lowering extra body fat, regular exercise helps people maintain a healthy weight. Retaining a healthy weight may help reduce the chance of developing several malignancies, including prostate, colon, and breast cancer.

Hormone Regulation: Physical activity has a role in controlling hormone levels, such as insulin and estrogen, which may impact the proliferation of cancer cells. Hormone-related malignancies may be less common in those with balanced hormone levels.

2. Boosting Immune Response

Increasing Immunity: Exercise regularly helps strengthen the immune system, making the body more resilient to infections and perhaps lowering the risk of certain malignancies by boosting immune surveillance against aberrant cells.

3. Encouraging Bone Health

Encouraging Digestion: Exercise promotes regular bowel movements and a healthy digestive system, which may lower the risk of colon cancer by reducing the amount of time that possible carcinogens remain in touch with the colon lining.

4. Handling Irritation

Mitigating Prolonged Inflammation: Prolonged inflammation has been linked to a higher chance of developing cancer. Through the stimulation of the body's anti-inflammatory reactions, exercise helps reduce chronic inflammation.

5. Effect on Particular Cancers

Breast Cancer: Research indicates that regular exercise may reduce the risk of breast cancer, particularly in youth and adulthood.

Colon Cancer: Studies have shown that physical activity may lower the incidence of colon cancer, especially for those who exercise moderately to vigorously regularly.

Suggested Exercise Protocols

Type: It is beneficial to engage in both strength training with weights or resistance bands and cardiovascular workouts like brisk walking, jogging, and cycling.

Duration: Try to get in 150 minutes or more of moderate-to-intense activity every week, spaced out across 75 minutes of strenuous exercise.

Consistency: The greatest health advantages come from long-term, consistent exercise routines.

Adaptation: Exercise programs must be customized based on each person's preferences and degree of fitness.

Vitamins and Supplements to Enhance Alkalinity

Although eating foods that are alkaline is the main goal of an alkaline diet, several vitamins and supplements may help support the body's efforts to become more alkaline. Some vitamins and supplements that are often linked to promoting alkalinity include the following:

First, vitamin C

Ascorbic Acid: Despite being acidic by nature, vitamin C-rich or citrus-based supplements may have alkalizing properties. They may boost immunological activity and improve general health.

Magnesium 2.

Glycinate or magnesium citrate: Supplements containing magnesium may help support several body processes and maintain the pH balance. They are often used to increase alkalinity and control the body's acidity levels.

Third, Powdered Greens

<u>Blends that Alkalize:</u> Alkaline-forming components such as wheatgrass, barley grass, spirulina, and chlorella are often included in greens powders. These supplements are meant to provide a concentrated amount of nutrients and raise alkalinity.

4. Potassium Citrate

<u>Potassium Citrate:</u> Known as an alkaline mineral, potassium aids in maintaining the body's pH equilibrium. Potassium-rich supplements may maintain optimal hydration, promote alkalinity, and support nerve function.

Fifth: Calcium

<u>Calcium carbonate or citrate:</u> Although calcium is an alkaline supplement, its use is not generally advised for the exclusive purpose of increasing alkalinity. Their importance for bone health notwithstanding, they could marginally promote an alkaline atmosphere.

6. Supplements with Bicarbonate

Sodium Bicarbonate: Sodium bicarbonate and other bicarbonate supplements have a high alkaline content. Due to their potent alkalizing action, however, their usage has to be carefully monitored and maintained.

7. Green algae

Chlorophyll Supplements: As a component of green vegetation, chlorophyll is often taken as a supplement. It is said to support the body's alkalinity and detoxifying processes.

8. Vitamin D

Vitamin D3: Although it has nothing to do with alkalinity, keeping enough of this vitamin in the body is vital for general health. The body's natural equilibrium may be indirectly supported by vitamin D supplementation.

Crucial Points to Remember:

A licensed dietician or other healthcare practitioner should be consulted before beginning any supplement plan to ascertain individual requirements and prevent possible interactions with drugs or medical conditions.

Balanced Approach: Supplements should not take the place of entire meals; rather, they should enhance a diet rich in foods that generate an alkaline state.

Although these supplements could help to promote alkalinity, a well-rounded diet rich in foods that generate an alkaline environment should still be the focus of one's diet. A wide variety of fruits, vegetables, nuts, seeds, and whole grains should be given priority as the main source of alkalinity support.

Conclusion

We have learned a great deal about the complex link between pH balance, nutrition, and general health as we have read through the pages of this in-depth reference to the alkaline diet and its possible influence on cancer defense.

We've explored the science behind pH balance, cellular health, and the complex relationships between nutrition and illness, from comprehending the fundamentals of the alkaline diet to learning about its possible involvement in cancer prevention. The study of alkaline foods and their advantages has brought to light the need to include nutrient-dense, plant-based foods in our diets.

Furthermore, we've discovered how crucial it is to make complimentary lifestyle adjustments and realized that an alkaline diet is just one aspect of the whole picture. Exercise, stress reduction strategies, and mindful living are all essential to promoting overall well-being.

When considering how vitamins and supplements might improve alkalinity, we have stressed the need for balance and consultation, keeping in mind that these additions should be used in conjunction with a diet high in whole, alkaline-forming foods rather than as a substitute for it.

As we get to the end of our trip, it is important to recognize that the alkaline diet is a useful strategy for promoting a better lifestyle rather than a miracle cure. The best way to fully reap its potential advantages for cancer prevention and general health is to combine it with mindful eating, consistent exercise, stress reduction, and a holistic approach to wellbeing.

Use this manual as a springboard for a more knowledgeable and thoughtful approach to nutrition, well-being, and vigor. May it enable you to live a life full of energy and well-being, adopt a diet rich in foods that generate an alkaline environment, and include holistic practices. All of these things contribute to possible cancer defense.

Date........,/....../.........

ingredient

note

Description

prep time: cook time:

Date.........../......./.........

Recipe Title:

ingredient

note

Description

prep time.   cook time.

Date........,/....../.........

Recipe Title:

ingredient

note

Description

prep time: cook time:

Date........./......./.........

ingredient

note

Description

prep time.   cook time.

Date............/........./...........

ingredient

note

Description

prep time: cook time:

Date........./......./.........

Recipe Title:

ingredient

note

Description

prep time: cook time:

Date........./......./.........

ingredient

note

Description

prep time: cook time:

Date........./......./.........

Recipe Title:

ingredient

note

Description

prep time.   cook time.

www.ingramcontent.com/pod-product-compliance
Lightning Source LLC
Chambersburg PA
CBHW070940260726
48661CB00003B/1060